INTERNAL
CLEANSING

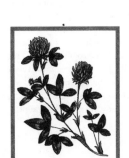

RID YOUR

BODY OF

TOXINS

AND RETURN

TO VIBRANT

GOOD HEALTH

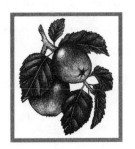

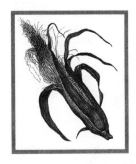

LINDA BERRY

PRIMA PUBLISHING

PRIMA PUBLISHING and colophon are registered trademarks of Prima Communications, Inc.

Disclaimer

Prima Publishing has designed this book to provide information in regard to the subject matter covered. It is sold with the understanding that the publisher and the author are not liable for the misconception or misuse of information provided. Every effort has been made to make this book as complete and as accurate as possible. The purpose of this book is to educate. The author and Prima Publishing shall have neither liability nor responsibility to any person or entity with respect to any loss, damage, or injury caused or alleged to be caused directly or indirectly by the information contained in this book. The information presented herein is in no way intended as a substitute for medical counseling.

All products mentioned in this book are trademarks of their respective companies.

Library of Congress Cataloging-in-Publication Data

Berry, Linda.
      Internal cleansing: rid your body of toxins and return to vibrant good health / Linda Berry.
          p.   cm.
      Includes bibliographical references and index.
      ISBN 0-7615-0859-7
      1. Toxicology—Popular works.   2. Health.   I. Title.
RA1213.B47   1997
613—dc21   97-3428
                                                                          CIP
          99 00 01 02 HH 10 9 8 7 6 5 4
Printed in the United States of America

Safe alternatives for household cleaning products, pages 71–73, reprinted, by permission, from *Creative Reuse Extravaganza*, developed by Project Create of the East Bay Depot for Creative Reuse, Inc., 6713 San Pablo Avenue, Oakland, CA 94608, 510-547-4733.

How to Order

Single copies may be ordered from Prima Publishing, P.O. Box 1260BK, Rocklin, CA 95677; telephone (916) 632-4400. Quantity discounts are also available. On your letterhead, include information concerning the intended use of the books and the number of books you wish to purchase.

Visit us online at http://www.primapublishing.com

This book is dedicated to you, the reader, in acknowledgment of your pursuit of better health. As we recognize the need for self-improvement and take steps in that direction, we also improve the health of our families, our communities, and the planet on which we live. In so doing, we honor the force that gives us life. Congratulations on your efforts!

It is generally not the disease but ignorance or neglect of the remedy which undermines the quality of one's life.

— *Mark Percival, D.C., N.D.,*
founder of Health Coach Systems International, Inc.

CONTENTS

FOREWORD

Through my 25 years in medical practice and health care as well as my personal and professional experience in juice fasting and detoxification, I have come to believe that the cleansing/detoxification process is the missing link in Western nutrition and one of the keys to real healing. I have seen hundreds of patients over the years transform regular or persistent illness into health and greatly improved vitality.

When we embark upon a purification process we instinctively take more time for ourselves and make our health a higher priority, whereby we are inspired to reevaluate our life, activities, habits, relationships, and more. We are then motivated to make new goals for our future. These goals usually involve making habit changes, such as letting go of daily abuses of sugar, caffeine, alcohol, nicotine, and junk foods. We also are inspired and guided to make decisions and take actions that we have sensed important but about which we had procrastinated or made excuses. Now we feel clear and present enough to make these changes in our work and career, home, relationships, and health.

One of my favorite experiences in medical practice is when I see the many positive side effects of natural therapies, especially from the cleansing process. Some of these wonderful side effects include reducing symptoms, elevating energy and attitude, and looking and feeling younger. I also receive many letters from readers who follow the guidelines in my books and experience improved health and many other positive changes in their lives.

More specifically, some of the medical concerns that I believe are related to toxicity and which respond well to detoxification are: allergies, arthritis, elevated cholesterol, high blood pressure, fatigue and sluggishness, backaches, body pains, and gastrointestinal disorders. In reality, most of the medical problems that take many years to develop and which we often label as chronic degenerative diseases respond well to cleansing therapies, as well as other natural therapies and lifestyle modifications.

Dr. Linda Berry offers us a fresh, clear voice in her simple, practical purification guidebook, *Internal Cleansing.* Dr. Berry first helps us to understand the many areas of potential stress in our lives and the problems that may occur; then she helps to orient us to the many things we can do, with lifestyle and natural therapies to help alleviate stress and clean and clear our body from the inside out. Linda also provides many practical references for us to pursue further knowledge and support from her many helpful guidelines.

I recommend this book highly as a useful guide to improving health and not just treating symptoms or disease. Since I believe that cleansing the body and mind is a process crucial to long-term health with vitality, and a key way to attain and maintain health for the 21st century, we must be aware of sources of toxicity that surround us so we can protect ourselves from them. *Internal Cleansing* by Dr. Linda Berry provides us with the beginning steps and long-range guidance by helping us to be informed and gives us the how-to's to reach for that next level of health and our optimal potential.

ELSON M. HAAS, M.D.

Dr. Elson M. Haas is the founder and medical director of the *Preventive Medical Center of Marin,* an integrated health care facility in San Rafael, California. He is also the author of four popular health books, including the highly acclaimed *Staying Healthy with the Seasons, Staying Healthy with Nutrition,* and his latest book, *The Detox Diet.*

ACKNOWLEDGMENTS

Many people have been instrumental in the formation of this book. I would especially like to thank Peter, Ryan, Mark, Cheri, Rita, Kathy, Jeff, Barb, Barbara, Melissa, Dr. Lukaczer, Tim, Bill, Dr. May, Juanita, Sandra, and Gary for your assistance, encouragement and/or resources. Thank you to all of my patients who have taught and inspired me with your quest for health. And thanks also to Skip, my beloved, for helping me with your vast array of knowledge and general life support. And finally, I would like to thank the divine from which all of this begins.

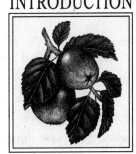

DO YOU NEED INTERNAL CLEANSING?

Each of us has within us the power to heal our pain and dysfunctions. In my years of practice as a doctor of chiropractic and five years as a Health Coach (see "What Is Health Coach?" page xvi), I have come to understand life as a balance of forces. Your daily choices determine your stress load. As you improve your lifestyle and minimize your negative reaction to stress, you increase your internal resilience and consequently improve your health and well-being.

Our bodies are the temples of our souls, and as such they deserve kind attention. Too often we neglect our health, placing our job, family, clients, and even our pets before ourselves. Instead of caring for ourselves and nourishing our body/mind/spirit, we often stuff ourselves full of harmful influences that can lead to blockage and congestion within our system. A safe, simple, and effective way to begin transforming negative, constipated energies is to cleanse your body so that it may serve rather than hinder your mind and soul, and cease interfering with your life's work.

Some people are motivated by pain, others are motivated by pleasure. What motivates you? If you don't change what you are doing now, your health will probably not improve. If you do make healthy changes, you will certainly feel better and you may even start feeling great.

I believe that an overburdened elimination system is the most common cause of ill health today, and the most dangerous. Fortunately, it is also treatable. In the words of one patient who once relied on laxatives (which treat only symptoms), "I have a chronic colon condition that causes a 'lazy colon.' I've spent fortunes on laxatives that really didn't work. With my doctor's permission, I started a colon cleansing program. I've been on it for seven weeks and I feel great." This patient benefited from a genuine cleansing program that addressed the causes of her ill health.

Looking at the big picture, I believe we are being cheated out of good health by ignorance. We live in a polluted environment, and our diet and lifestyle make us prone to chronic illness. Understanding that our quality of life is determined by our daily choices, we have the power to improve our health and well-being step by step. With the proper use of cleansing, we can keep our bodies healthy and vital, even as we age. Chronic ailments that are believed to be a natural part of aging can be halted in their tracks and often reversed by using health practices that take only a few moments each day. In this book, you will find simple, practical, and effective methods to help your body function as it was designed to.

Do You Need Internal Cleansing?

Our bodies perform internal cleansing on a daily, moment-by-moment basis. But our normal channels of detoxification can be overwhelmed by the polluted environment in which we live, a food supply laden with pesticides and preservatives and deficient in nutrients due to mineral-depleted soil, and an internal milieu of toxic residue caused by drugs and the by-products of a stressful life. Our natural cleansing processes need our help.

You can assist the normal cleansing process most effectively by decreasing your stress load and engaging in periodic cleansing programs (I will use the words "detoxification" and "cleansing" interchangeably in this book). Chapters 1, 4, 5, and 6 will help you identify the keys areas of stress that contribute to failing health. Chapter 2 identifies how food and toxins are processed by your body and Chapter 3 describes the five necessities for healthy bowel action. Chapter 6 discusses environmental toxins and how they affect you. Chapters 8, 9, and 10 introduce you to three cleansing programs: the first one involves food only; the second employs herbal and fiber products that can be purchased in your health food store; and the third involves a shift in what you eat, moving away from the most common food allergens while introducing scientifically formulated and proven therapeutic food powders. This third program must be carried out with the support of a licensed health care practitioner. All of the recommended cleansing programs take approximately eight weeks to complete.

For those of you who want to support cleansing without engaging in a specific program, you will find recommendations throughout *Internal Cleansing,* and specifically in Chapters 7, 11, 12, 13, 14, and 15.

Before I explain the details of cleansing programs that I recommend, you should look over the following checklist to determine whether you would benefit from internal cleansing. Then complete the Metabolic Screening Questionnaire and the Dysbiosis Questionnaire in Chapter 8 to assess your health status. These tools will give you an idea of whether you have toxic buildup in your body.

Autointoxication Checklist

If you experience any of the following symptoms, you may be experiencing *autointoxication* (a process whereby you are poisoned by substances produced by your own body as a result of inadequate digestion and elimination), and therefore you might want to consider some type of internal cleansing program.

- allergy or intolerance to certain foods
- bad breath and foul-smelling gas and stools
- constipation, diarrhea, sluggish elimination, irregular bowel movements
- frequent congestion, colds, viruses
- flatulence or gas and frequent intestinal disorders
- frequent headaches for no apparent reason
- general aches and pains that migrate from one place to another
- intolerance to fatty foods
- low energy; loss of vitality for no apparent reason
- lower back pain
- lowered resistance to infections

- needing to sleep a long time
- pain in your liver or gall bladder
- premenstrual syndrome (PMS), breast soreness, vaginal infections
- skin problems, rashes, boils, pimples, acne

If you have severe symptoms or any serious disorders, seek the attention of a competent health care provider. The above list is only meant to indicate some of the symptoms of autointoxication. Anyone who has been on a Standard American Diet (SAD) for more than two years would benefit from periodic cleansing, especially if you live in an urban area.

Please note that pregnant or lactating women should postpone their cleansing program, as toxic substances can be released to the fetus during cleansing, through the shared circulation of the mother's blood or through the mother's milk. If you are pregnant or lactating, you can still help yourself and your little one by eating high-quality food and supplementing your diet with fiber and other health promoting nutrients as described in Chapter 13. Following the general rule of five servings of fruits and vegetables and one whole grain each day will support your special needs, along with essential fatty acids, rest, prenatal vitamins, and an increased consumption of water (see Appendix 2 on Infant Care).

WHERE TO START

Any cleansing program should begin by "pulling the plug" that blocks the passage of waste. The "plug" is in your colon, the last portion of your food-processing chain. If you try to clean your blood, lymph, or liver without first addressing a stopped-up large intestine, the excreted toxins will get right back into your body and make you sicker than you were before you started.

A carefully planned and monitored cleansing program will not make you sick. It has the potential to make you feel gloriously better. Sometimes just by freeing up your intestines, you can reduce the need for cleansing other circulatory or organ systems. Removing the reservoir of poisons downstream prevents them from accumulating upstream.

If you took your heart or lung cells and put them in a laboratory dish, giving the cells the food they need to live and washing away their waste products, your cells would outlive you because they would be provided with an optimum environment. When you have finished reading this book, you will have the information you need to nourish and cleanse all of your cells, creating a more optimal environment in order to begin a more healthful, positive way of living.

WHAT IS HEALTH COACH?

Some would have us believe that health is the mere absence of disease. The World Health Organization (WHO) defines health as the presence of complete social, mental, and physical well-being, not merely the absence of disease. Health Coach Systems International takes that definition a step farther: "Health is that state of mind, body, and spirit that allows for proper function, joy, and peace of mind." Health Coach, founded in 1991 by Mark Percival, D.C., N.D., is a group of over 200 licensed heath care practitioners in North America from various fields, who use education, inspiration, and natural therapies to help their clients and patients overcome pain, fatigue, and illness to achieve radiant health. According to Health Coach, there are four fundamental aspects of health:

1. Rest/movement/exercise
2. Eating appropriately
3. Self-reflection
4. Fun/community or loving relationships

Creating these essentials in your life is what Health Coach calls "no alternative" or self-reliant health care. No alternative simply means that there is no alternative to

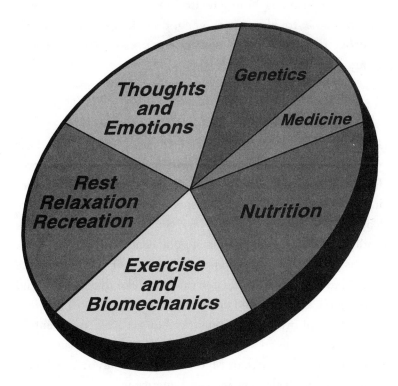

What Determines Your Health

As you can see, your lifestyle choices are the greatest influence on your health. Education is the foundation of your healthcare, and with better education you make better choices.

(Reprinted by permission of Health Coach Systems International, Inc., and New Health Perspectives.)

drinking good water, thinking good thoughts, getting rest, moving your body, eating good food, and having fun. By taking care of these fundamentals you will enjoy vibrant good health.

Take a moment to reflect on these four fundamentals and notice that they are influenced by your daily choices and actions. The quality of your life is determined by the quality of your choices. Of course, genetics plays a role in your health. Take a look at the chart on page xvii to see "What Determines Your Health." At the present time, it is not possible to alter your genetic makeup, but you can improve the way your genetic code expresses itself by modifying your daily lifestyle choices.

AWARENESS + ACTION = HEALTH

Health is your birthright. You can educate yourself about how your body works, and/or seek the help of a trained health professional, and begin to make wiser, health-promoting choices in the realms of eating, exercise, relaxation, and relationship, leading to a happier, healthier you. Start with some baby steps until you can take the pursuit of your health into a full-blown, joyous gallop. As British statesman and orator Edmund Burke said, "No one would make a greater mistake than he who did nothing because he could do only a little."

One of my patients remarked to me after treatment, "I have just completed six weeks of the internal cleansing program and feel better than I have in years—maybe ever! This is something I feel everyone can benefit by."

It is my hope that you, too, will feel the same way soon.

PART I:
NEEDS AND REMEDIES AN OVERVIEW

CHAPTER 1

FOUR KINDS OF STRESS

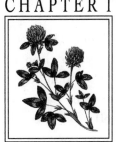

Faced with adversity, human beings show an amazing ability to adapt. So why do we break down with symptoms of ill health and disease? The answer is that we encounter or endure stress greater than our body/mind can handle.

Four major kinds of stress lead to dysfunction, disease, and death: structural stress, biochemical stress, mental and emotional stress, and electromagnetic stress. Stress causes an accumulation of toxic substances and waste products in your system. Each thought, emotion, or physical action you take evokes a physiological biochemical state in your body. Toxic thoughts and emotions such as hatred, impatience, or fear create toxic chemicals with harmful effects in your body. The physical trauma of accidents or repetitive stress may result in an overproduction of internally produced chemicals that prove harmful to your system. A key Health Coach principle to keep in mind is: "The single greatest challenge your body faces is the effective management of toxins." How can this be

3

done? The main focus of this book is to offer a variety of ways to clean up the toxic waste dump that is almost certainly building up in your body with the stressors of each passing day. *Internal Cleansing* will guide you to proven and effective therapies to remove obstacles that are interfering with your effective detoxification and elimination pathways. Here you'll find simple, inexpensive, and effective procedures to decrease your toxic stress load.

To handle short-term stress situations, your body moves into an alarm state. Your adrenal glands secrete hormones that shut down the supply of blood to your muscles, make you breathe faster and more shallowly, make your heart pump stronger and faster, and increase your sensory awareness. The long-term stress of a fast-paced life, filled with problems that nag you daily without resolution, also creates this alarm state on a chronic low-level basis. This depletes your energy and your adrenal glands, ruins your digestion, and takes a toll on your health and peace of mind. Because your body does not have the opportunity to rebound between stressful moments with rest, relaxation, or exercise, you have little chance to replenish your energy reserves.

Dr. Kenneth Pelletier, a psychologist from the University of California School of Medicine in San Francisco, has found that the body cannot tell the difference between a "real" threat and an imagined one. So the potential stressful situations that you worry about every day are as harmful to your physiology as the actual stress you face. All of these underlying worries translate into damage to your body. Japanese researchers found that mental stress changed the environment in the intestinal tract to favor the growth of pathogenic microbes at the expense of health-promoting bacteria. Why not replace worry with positive action?

More than twenty-five years ago, public health officials noticed an epidemic increase in the number of heart and blood-vessel diseases, which prompted an intensive search for the cause. Their discoveries placed the responsibility on dietary issues: increased intake of fat and sugar, and decreased intake of fiber. Several characteristics of the Western lifestyle were also significant factors, including a reduced level of physical exertion at work and at home, reliance on legal drugs such as alcohol and nicotine for relaxation and caffeine for a pick-me-up, and most importantly the increased stresses linked to a fast paced, ever changing pattern of life. All of these stressors have been medically documented as contributing to a widespread increase in chronic degenerative illness and reduced overall health.

STRUCTURAL STRESS

Structural stress begins with birth. Newborns are often pulled forcibly out of the mother's womb. Some are grabbed with metal forceps or sucked out of the birth canal with a metal cap attached to the head. Nor does a cesarean delivery ensure a gentle birth. The doctor pulls on the head, the shoulder—whatever can be grabbed as the baby emerges. A medical technician whom I know saw doctors in the emergency room brace their feet against the delivery table as they yanked the baby out. This is not a good beginning for your musculoskeletal and nervous systems.

Structural stress continues as you grow up and through adulthood. How many times have you fallen, been hit with a ball, or gotten knocked down in a game of basketball, baseball, football, or volleyball? How many times have you strained your back or the joints in your arms and legs while playing tennis or golf, or fallen off your bicycle, or hit the ground while rollerblading? Sports are fun *and* they can cause physical blows that lead to physical damage. Not to mention the automobile accidents you may have encountered, or the injuries sustained while being a home fix-it person. Even going to the dentist causes structural stress because of the head and mouth positions you must maintain while having work done on your teeth and gums. Many of my patients are coming in these days with repetitive stress injuries from their desk jobs. Sitting and working in a limited space and performing a limited number of motions are very confining for the body and contribute to muscular stress. Desk work may put significant harmful strain on your lower back, wrists, hands, forearms, shoulders, and neck.

More commonly, people can be structurally stressed by the quality of the food that they eat. A male patient in his thirties came in one day complaining of pain in his back in the area just below his shoulder blades. He had a *subluxation* (misalignment) of one of the vertebra in that area, and after a chiropractic adjustment and rubbing reflexes associated with the small intestines that run along the bottom edge of the ribcage he was pain-free. I found out that he had just returned from a trip, and the airplane food he had eaten had not sat well in his system. As a result, the nerves in his small intestines became irritated, which then "short-circuited" his spine and caused the misalignment. The small intestine reflex was probably activated by congestion in his gastrointestinal (GI) system from the less-than-optimal food he had eaten.

BIOCHEMICAL STRESS

Biochemical stress is becoming an increasingly common cause of ill health, leading to chronic ill health and death. Our government has known for a long time that we are exposed to many dangerous compounds. The U.S. government's Special Commission of 1977:369 stated, "What cannot be overlooked are the unknown consequences—among them the teratogenic and conceivably mutagenic effects—of the unremitting barrage of chemicals to which the populations of the industrialized world are subjected." (*Teratogenic* means "causing developmental malformations," and *mutagenic* means "inducing genetic mutation.") There are now over 60,000 synthetic chemicals being produced commercially, and about 1,000 newly synthesized compounds are introduced each year—that's nearly *three new chemicals per day*. These chemicals come in the form of drugs (over-the-counter, recreational, and prescription), food additives, pesticides, fuels, chemical fertilizers, household cleaners, glues, solvents, and by-products of industry that are released into the environment. As early as 1977, our government has been concerned about the harmful effects of manmade chemicals, but not enough has been done to protect the public.

The outside world is not the only source of toxins that disturb your health. Toxins are also produced inside your body by improper digestion of food. Before you say, "That's not me; I digest my food just fine," pause for a moment to recall if you have ever experienced gas in your intestines. Many people deal with gas on a regular basis. These gurgling and sometimes embarrassing vapors are the work of bacteria or yeasts gobbling up undigested food particles in your small and large intestines. These particles result from improper food combinations, from eating foods that your body does not agree with, and/or from eating in a rushed or agitated emotional state. (Chapter 2 examines what happens in a healthy gut and how the gut malfunctions.)

Chronically fatigued and immune-compromised people from my practice found that avoiding substances toxic to them was the most significant step they had taken to reclaim their health. Although you cannot totally avoid environmental pollutants, you can improve your ability to transform toxins into harmless materials. These converted poisons can then be safely eliminated through your normal excretory channels of sweat, urine, feces, and breath. (Chapter 3 describes ways to enhance your ability to eliminate toxins.)

If your body cannot remove toxins through normal excretion (its first line of defense), it will take stepped-up measures to protect itself. This is when you begin to get the "itises": colitis, sinusitis, gastritis, bronchitis, and appendicitis, to name just a few. Terms like "bronchitis," "gastritis," and others generally denote an inflammation of the part to which the ending -itis is attached. Inflammation is your body's second line of healing defense—a way of healing itself by killing off foreign invaders such as germs and allergens, diluting injurious substances such as toxins, walling off a problem area to prevent it from spreading, or simply stabilizing a weakened or injured area. When your second line of defense is ineffective at expelling waste, toxins begin to accumulate in your body in polyps, cysts, and tumors, which can progress to cancer.

ELECTROMAGNETIC STRESS

Electromagnetic stress is everywhere, from radios, televisions, cellular phones, radar, and microwaves. Young children and electrical workers are especially vulnerable to these energy frequencies. Although this is a controversial topic, research from the late 1970s through the 1990s supports a closer look at exposure to electromagnetic fields (EMFs). Swedish studies from 1993 show a higher incidence of leukemia in children who live near high voltage power lines (*American Journal of Epidemiology*, 1993). Electrical workers show a significantly increased risk of leukemia and central-nervous-system-related tumors (*American Industrial Hygiene Association Journal*, 1993). Exposure can also come from electrical appliances, including televisions (sitting too close to televisions increases your exposure to electrical radiation; protect children by making a minimum distance rule while they watch television—at least three feet from the screen) and cooking appliances, and from electrically conductive plumbing (*Bioelectromagnetics*, 1995). Electrically conductive plumbing is found in homes whose electricity is grounded to their water pipes in an uninterrupted metallic path to the water main which is also connected to neighboring houses. To find out if your home's electricity is grounded in this manner, you can call your local building inspector. Alternative grounding options exist. The grounding wire for your house can be connected to a nine to ten foot copper rod buried in the ground anywhere outside your home.

We are on electromagnetic overload. Mark Percival, D.C., N.D., tells about one of his patients who suffered from nightly seizures that were not relieved by medication. After carefully reviewing his case, Dr. Percival offered a number of options to decrease the stressors to this man's health and to increase his internal resilience. The patient's first steps were to increase his exposure to natural light by going outside on breaks, setting up a filter screen which reduces radiation exposure for his computer monitor, and moving his LED (light emitting diode) clock from his bedside across the room to his dresser. After only one day, this man's nighttime seizures went away. It pays to take a serious look at reducing your exposure to potentially harmful electromagnetic frequencies.

MENTAL/EMOTIONAL STRESS

At my office, we have learned to appreciate the effects of state of mind on health. Often we see patients with pain between their shoulder blades or in the area between their neck and shoulder who reveal a deep anger or hurt they have been holding inside. Their pain subsides when they work through this emotion and transform it or find constructive ways to dissipate the tension they created from their repressed feelings. Anger may also cause pain and/or weakness in different parts of your body. In the Applied Kinesiology (AK) system of diagnosis and treatment (borrowing from the Chinese Five Element healing system), the pectoral muscle in your chest relates to the liver. Liver function is disturbed by anger. When people get angry they sometimes experience chest pain, which may be mistaken for a heart problem.

Knee pain may also relate to liver dysfunction; the *popliteus* muscle, which nestles into the back of your knee, is another muscle that relates to the liver in the AK system. Several years ago, a woman came to my office with pain in her knees. Her mother had just died, and she was afraid that she, too, was falling apart. Upon examination, I found that the popliteus muscle behind her knee and the reflexes associated with her liver were involved. Problems in these areas can be associated with anger. I asked if she had been angry recently, and she said she had. Her mother was an alcoholic who had left a mess of her home and her affairs, which my patient had to straighten out. She was angry at her mother for being an alcoholic, for dying with complications of alcoholism, *and* for leaving such a mess for her to take care of. Just knowing that her emotions were involved in her knee pain gave this patient a sense of relief. We worked on the involved areas, and she left feeling much better and had no more trouble with her knees.

Lower back pain frequently results from a disturbance of bowel function precipitated by an emotional upset or trauma. Handle the emotional upset, and the irritation carried by the nerves to the digestive organs is eliminated or decreased.

Sharon Wegscheider-Cruse, a psychologist who has been writing about dysfunctional family relationships since 1987, estimates that ninety-six percent of us are raised in dysfunctional families (source: Sharon Wegscheider-Cruse). Most of us were not raised in homes that nourished growth or supported confidence and self-esteem. Linda G. Russek and Gary E. Schwartz, in "Narrative Descriptions of Parental Love and Caring Predict Health Status in Midlife: A 35-Year Follow-Up of the Harvard Mastery of Stress Study" from the Harvard publication *Alternative Therapies* (November 1996), state: "The perception of social support is reportedly a significant predictor of future health." Students from the 1950s were asked at that time to write narrative descriptions of their parents. They found that subjects who had illnesses in mid-life such as coronary artery disease, hypertension, duodenal ulcer, and alcoholism had used significantly fewer positive words such as *loving, friendly, warm, open, understanding, sympathetic,* and *just* to describe their parents. Furthermore, ninety-five percent of subjects who used few positive words and who also rated their parents low in parental caring had diseases diagnosed in mid-life, whereas only twenty-nine percent of subjects who used many positive words and also rated their parents high in parental caring had these problems. The effect was independent of the subject's age, family history of illness, smoking behavior, marital history, or the death or divorce of the subject's parents.

Emotional traumas accumulate early and may persist, leaving a person with emotional scars that get carried into adult life and relationships. To add further insult to injury, much inner dialogue is negative. In *Over the Top*, Zig Ziglar says, "The most important opinion you have is the one you have of yourself, and the most significant things you say are those things you say to yourself." One of my mentors, Charles Ward, D.C., founder of Legends in Leadership, a practice management organization, likes to remind his audience that if anyone talked to us the way we talk to ourselves we would want to get away from that person as fast as possible. Self-destructive inner dialogue may be limiting your ability to take positive steps to heal your life and your health. (For action steps you can take to resolve such internal conflicts see Appendix 1.)

Stress of all kinds wears your body down and leads to an increased toxic burden in one of two ways.

1. By depleting your energy reserves and nutrients necessary for normal elimination.
2. By causing an increase in toxic metabolites as a result of negative thoughts, moods and emotions, physical trauma, and impaired digestive capacity.

Keep reading. You will find solutions to the problem of toxic buildup in the following pages.

CHAPTER 2

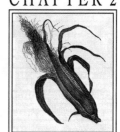

How the Body Processes Food and Toxins

The Digestive Process

In order to survive and thrive, your body must change the products you eat into microparticles which, when absorbed, move into place to nourish your cells and become the components of your body. This process is called digestion and assimilation, or absorption. You may have heard the expression "You are what you eat." Actually, you are what you absorb. The intricate workings of your digestive system are dependent on mechanical action such as chewing and peristalsis, and on biochemical responses such as the secretion of enzymes. If one facet of digestion is malfunctioning, or if nutritional mediators are absent, the end products of eating become hazardous to your health, as you will learn in this chapter.

How Digestion Works

The chemical process of digestion begins when the thought or smell of food causes secretion of a starch-metabolizing enzyme in your saliva. Perhaps you have noticed how the simple act of talking about food can make you feel hungry.

IN THE MOUTH   Mechanical action, or chewing, is the next step. Chewing is also known as *mastication*. At the turn of the century, an American food scientist named Horace Fletcher went public with the importance of chewing. He encouraged folks to "Fletcherize" their food. The process was simple: chew each bite about fifty times and ingest liquids by sips.

The chemical phase of digestion begins in earnest after mouthfuls of food have been broken down by chewing. If you gulp food down in big bites without much chewing, you put the brakes on your ability to digest food and be well-nourished because digestive juices will not come in contact with all parts of the food you have swallowed.

In the mouth, the chemical process is initiated with the release of *ptyalin*, an enzyme that begins carbohydrate (starch) digestion. You can taste the results of this enzyme's activity if you take a cracker, a piece of plain bread, or a bite of plain pasta and chew it until you get a sweet taste in your mouth. A carbohydrate is made up of individual sucrose (sugar) molecules. The sweet taste comes from the conversion of the starch in the cracker, bread, or pasta into simple sugars. This may be a good way for you to judge if you are chewing your food enough: wait until the carbohydrates in your mouth become sweet from adequate chewing before swallowing.

IN THE STOMACH   In the stomach, hydrochloric acid acts as a bulldozer and further breaks up large food particles into a semiliquid called *chyme*. Peristalsis aids the mixing of the chyme with digestive secretions to enhance the complete breakdown of food. Finally, the real digestive finesse begins: enzymes released from the pancreas and gallbladder, called amylase, lipase, and protease, divide carbohydrates, fats, and proteins into simple sugars, fatty acids, and amino acids, respectively. The first portion of the small intestine, called the duodenum, is where the last phase of enzyme production is completed.

IN THE SMALL INTESTINE   Absorption occurs primarily in the upper portion of the small intestine. There is, however, significant absorption of key nutrients in the colon, specifically the B-vitamins. When you were growing in your mother's womb, your body formed special surfaces in your intestinal tract for nutrient absorption. These surfaces are called *villi*. In the small intestine, you have even smaller finger-like projections called *microvilli* that extend into your gut lumen (the enclosed space within your intestinal tract). The microvilli are hair-like projections that carry lymphatic and blood vessels to your gut wall to interface with the partially digested food you have recently eaten. (See "How Poor Digestion Affects the Lymphatic System," page 27.) It takes approximately twenty minutes for food to clear your stomach and reach this digestive station. Peristaltic movement makes it possible for the chyme to wash against the absorptive surfaces of the microvilli. The gut lumen and the lung tissue have the highest concentration of protective immune cells in the body because both areas come in contact with potentially contaminating substances such as are found in food and in the air.

What is finally absorbed from the intricate processes of your digestive system are simple sugars from carbohydrates, amino acids from proteins, and fatty acids from fats. All of these macronutrients (protein, carbohydrates, fat) which appear in food are essential for life. Macronutrients must be broken down into microparticles before they can be absorbed.

IN THE COLON   The colon, the last portion of your digestive system, is the final treatment area for whatever enters the digestive tract. Its job is to compact the chyme, absorb water, and receive B-vitamins that are produced by healthy intestinal bacteria. The bacteria in your intestines are called *intraluminal* cells. They are tiny particles much smaller than your body's cells, and they are packed in tightly. In fact, there are more individual cells in your intestinal tract than there are known stars in the universe.

The hundred or more strains of bacteria that coexist in the intestines can be thought of as a neighborhood. There are "good guys" ready to work for your health and "bad guys" out to eat up your good nutrients, poke holes in your intestines in search of more goodies, and scavenge food that has overstayed its welcome, forming dangerous chemical by-products. These "bad-guy" bacteria create toxic substances that further injure your intestinal wall, and eventually injure your joints, skin, organs, and endocrine glands. Such every-day problems as gas and bad breath are caused by these pathogenic microorganisms, but they can also create life-threatening diseases like cancer.

Digestive System Breakdown

If you are under stress or in a negative state of mind when you eat, your digestive system gets a message from your nervous system to shut down and take a break because the blood and energy used for digestion are needed elsewhere. If this happens, the fat that you eat becomes rancid, the carbohydrates ferment, and the proteins putrefy. This leads to bad breath, possibly indigestion, and altered bowel activity— either too much activity, causing loose stool, or too little, causing constipation. Instead of getting nutrients to feed your cells and create new ones, your cells get a serving of more waste to deal with. After a while, your cells can't handle any more waste and they begin to break down or malfunction.

Autointoxication is the process of the body poisoning itself with toxins, from internal sources, that cannot be processed by the body's elimination systems because they are overloaded, undernourished, genetically compromised, or diseased. If the organs of elimination are not functioning properly, the waste matter will not be eliminated and the toxic residue will be reabsorbed into the bloodstream, causing chronic unwellness and possibly disease.

A poorly functioning digestive tract can turn even the best of foods into metabolic poisons in the form of acids, gases, alcohols, and carcinogens. This kind of digestive trouble is becoming a major source of internal toxicity in many North Americans. The fastest and surest way to detoxify your system is through improving the quality of your digestion.

Health Consequences of Intestinal Irritants   The presence of pathogenic organisms in the gut has been linked to arthritic disorders. As reported in the *Archives of Surgery* (December 1988), trauma, burns, chemotherapy, and inflammatory bowel disease can be related to an increase in the permeability of your bowel to microorganisms or to their endotoxins (toxic by-products). This is a condition called "leaky gut." In *The Journal of Rheumatology* (December

1985), Smith, Gibson, and Brooks reported finding "significant alterations in bowel permeability in patients with ankylosing spondylitis (AS) and rheumatoid arthritis (RA). An association between bacterial flora in the bowel, diet, and intestinal mucosal permeability and joint disease in patients with RA and AS has been suggested by several authors and our study further links the GI tract and inflammatory joint disease."

Myasthenia gravis, a disease of the nerve/muscle junction, has been described as an *autoimmune disease*, which means that the body attacks its own cells. How does the body turn against itself? In *Medical Intelligence* (vol. 312, n. 4), Stefansson and others propose a model of infestation by pathogenic bacteria in the gut. The immune system reacts to the bacterial infestation. Unfortunately, in myasthenia gravis the nerve/muscle junction looks like pathogenic bacteria to the circulating immune system cells, so they attack the vital communication link between the nervous system and muscle function.

Marjatta Leirisal-Repo, M.D., and Heikki Repo, M.D., at the Second Department of Medicine at the University of Helsinki reported that infections of the mucosa—the lining of the inner ear and the digestive and elimination systems—can trigger the development of reactive arthritis. The infection can be in the urogenital tract (the tube going from your bladder to the outside of your body) or in the gastrointestinal (GI) tract. The microbes that most frequently triggered the arthritic response were chlamydia, shigella, salmonella, yersinia, and campylobacter. You may have heard from your doctor that the problems you were having in your elimination channels were caused by one or more of these microbes.

In an editorial in the *Journal of Rheumatology* (1987) by Inman, it is learned that many gastrointestinal problems are related to arthritis. People who have had intestinal bypass surgery, dysentery (Montezuma's Revenge), inflammatory bowel disease, parasites, colitis, and milk allergies plus other bowel disorders have a higher incidence of arthritis than people with normal GI tracts.

What these researchers are saying is that the pain you may be experiencing in your joints could be due to a toxic bowel, to allergies, or to an autoimmune response caused by a similarity between your cells and harmful microorganisms. Internal cleansing is a possible solution to these problems (for more information, see Chapters 7 and 8).

The standard medical solution for arthritis and joint pain is nonsteroidal anti-inflammatory drugs (NSAIDs), such as Tylenol, Motrin, acetaminophen, ibuprofen, and aspirin, generally available over the counter. If NSAIDs don't relieve the pain, sometimes a medical doctor will prescribe steroids. While NSAIDs and steroids usually provide temporary relief from aches and pains, most NSAIDs inhibit the liver's ability to neutralize toxic substances, thus causing an overload of toxins in the bloodstream. Formerly injured or painful areas then become further irritated by the toxins in the blood, which in turn renews the pain cycle.

Many people notice irritation to their digestive tract when using NSAIDs. These substances can actually cause the lining of the stomach and intestines to bleed. And like antibiotics that kill off both the good and the bad bacteria, NSAIDs kill off the natural pain-relieving substances that the body produces from the good fats and oils one eats. (As a chiropractic student, I was amazed to study the effects of steroid hormones on rat joints. I can still clearly see in my mind's eye a series of photomicrographs of a normal rat joint and its appearance after only two cortisone injections. After one injection, the distinct surfaces of the joint began to break down and bleed into each other. After the second injection the joint was completely obliterated. All of the cells had become non-distinct scar tissue instead of bone, carti-lage, and synovial cells. Seeing those photos made up my mind about ever getting a steroid injection.)

If you must use NSAIDs or steroids, it is wise to use them minimally and to seek effective treatment for the cause of your pain with a respected chiropractor. Also, follow the cleansing recommendations throughout this book to minimize or eliminate the inflammatory agents that trigger your pain.

FOOD AND HEALTH

There are five major or *macronutrient* categories required for life: water, proteins, carbohydrates, fats, and fiber. The cur-rent craze for a high-carbohydrate, lowfat diet is not com-patible with human physiology. We need approximately twenty to thirty percent good fats, twenty to thirty percent protein, and forty to sixty percent carbohydrates.

Because we are all biochemically individual, we each need different proportions of fats, protein, and carbohy-drates. Depending on what is happening in your life, your individual needs also change. If your diet consists mostly of refined carbohydrates such as pasta, crackers, and bread, you are creating an imbalance in your body that promotes fat storage, increases pain, suppresses your immune system, depletes your hormones, destabilizes your cell membranes, and places strain on your heart and blood vessels. Likely outcomes of this kind of diet include obesity; muscle and joint pains; increased susceptibility to infection, common colds, and flu; infertility, impotency, and menstrual difficulties; wrinkles, dry skin, and acne; and heart attacks and blood vessel disease.

The Vicious Cycle of Food Hypersensitivity

Many people were fed food other than their mother's milk as an infant, before their digestive tract had completely formed. In such people there is a high probability of food hypersensitivities. Think about the foods that babies are typically fed: cow's milk and related dairy products, cereal grains (especially wheat), eggs, citrus, and soy-based products. These are the most common food *allergens* (an allergen is a substance that causes a hypersensitive or allergic reaction). The high incidence of childhood ear infections (treated by one antibiotic after another and too often culminating in surgery to insert plastic tubes into the ears of preschool-age children) is probably the result of food hypersensitivities (see Appendix 1).

To add to your digestive confusion, grains have only been a part of the human diet for the past ten thousand years. That is a long time compared to the human life span but a very short time compared to the length of time that humans have inhabited the earth. In most native cultures people who eat grains sprout them before eating to make them more digestible and they culture milk products before use for the same reason. Other causes of food allergies are weakened adrenal glands from too much stress and inadequate times spent resting, relaxing, and exercising, and a weak or impaired digestive system from drugs, alcohol, antibiotics, excess sugar, preservatives, pesticides and food additives, lack of variety in the diet or eating the same foods over and over, and a deficiency of digestive enzyme secretion by your body.

If you are eating foods to which you are hypersensitive, you may suffer with fatigue, heart palpitations, insomnia, indigestion, the full component of digestive disturbances, frequent illnesses, confusion, mental disorders, body aches and pains; anything can go wrong. At a Health Coach Retreat called "Physician Heal Thyself," doctors and their support staff reintroduced foods after eliminating major food allergens for a six-day period and eating a simple diet. Upon reintroduction, reactions included anxiety from eating an egg; unrelenting diarrhea, an upper respiratory infection, and depression from eating wheat; burning pain running down the backs of both arms and legs from eating tomatoes; depression from eating brown rice; and lethargy from eating millet. If you eat a food to which you are hypersensitive every day, you won't have such a pronounced reaction. Instead of getting an acute attack of sickness, you will be chronically unwell; your body adapts to the substance.

STEROID USE AND FOOD HYPERSENSITIVITIES   If you have had a history of antibiotic or steroid use, including birth control pills and cortisone and its medical relatives—or even if you have drunk chlorinated water—the chances are good that you have an imbalance of intestinal microorganisms, with the bad guys outweighing the good guys. When this happens, the pathogenic yeasts or bacteria may invade or irritate your intestinal wall, causing damage that leads to a "leaky gut." The leaky gut allows big molecules of food to pass through your intestinal wall and enter your bloodstream. Your immune system is then put on alert and mobilizes lymphocytes, macrophages, natural killer cells, and the like to protect you against these foreign invaders to your bloodstream. An inflammatory cascade ensues which may lead to colitis, irritable bowel syndrome, sinusitis, arthritis, or any other -*itis* you can imagine.

How Food Combining Impacts Digestion

Some nutrition experts emphasize proper food combining to solve digestive upset. In brief, because of enzyme action, you digest your food more easily if you avoid eating starches and proteins in combination. (John Montague, Fourth Earl of Sandwich, started a lot of trouble with his eighteenth-century invention of putting meat between two slices of bread.) Most meals are nightmares of bad food combining— think about the Standard American Diet (SAD):

- Breakfast: Orange juice with simple sugars; toast, usually a refined carbohydrate with little fiber; eggs, a protein; and bacon, a protein/fat food full of carcinogenic nitrosamines.
- Lunch: Typically a sandwich or burger consisting of starch and protein.
- Dinner: More meat with potatoes or rice (starch and protein) and a sugar-rich dessert.

Eating this way causes several days' worth of meals to back up in your intestines (Figure 2.1). No wonder Americans have such upset stomachs after all!

If you have digestive complaints, first try eating your food in a more relaxed state of mind and spend more time eating your food. If that doesn't help, you might want to experiment with eating less food or with food-combining

Food transit time of person on a Standard American Diet (low fiber) diet. Average transit time is 65–100 hours.

Food transit time of person on a high fiber diet. Average transit time is 20–45 hours.

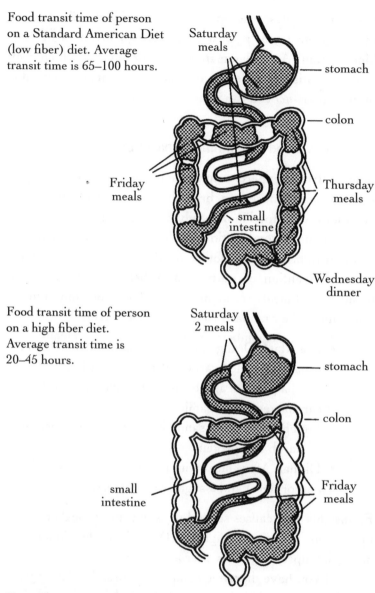

NOTE: The person on the Standard American Diet holds eight meals of undigested food and waste material in the colon, while the person on the high fiber diet holds only three.

Figure 2.1   Food Transit Times

principals. When you eat high-starch vegetables, combine them only with high-water-content vegetables (see "Carbohydrate Classifications of Fruits and Vegetables," Chapter 8). When you eat protein, combine it only with high-water-content vegetables. In practice, if you eat the bread that is served before your meal in a restaurant, you would choose a vegetable meal and eat your protein at a later time. Or avoid eating the bread and eat only the vegetables and protein on your plate, but not the rice or potatoes. I often ask for a double portion of vegetables instead of the starch on the menu when I eat a protein meal out. You may benefit from doing the same if you have digestive difficulties.

I find that my digestive system gets in an uproar if I eat raw fruit and raw vegetables at the same meal. You might also consider eating melons alone. Your digestive system is unique. Only by trial and error will you find the right food combinations. Remember: Awareness + Action = Health.

How the Thyroid Affects Digestion and Elimination

To have a healthy digestive tract, you must also have a properly functioning thyroid gland. Thyroid hormones help your intestines with peristalsis; if you have a sluggish thyroid, you will probably have a sluggish bowel, causing chronic constipation and the subsequent backup of toxins into your blood. Unfortunately, current blood tests for thyroid function only tell us the amount of thyroid hormone in your blood; they cannot tell us whether the hormone is getting into your cells and working where it's supposed to.

Thyroid blood tests are unreliable because we can't get information on the functional capacity of the thyroid from blood tests. Dr. Broda O. Barnes developed a protocol for evaluating the function of the thyroid gland by measuring underarm temperature *before* you get out of bed in the morning. You do this test with an old-fashioned thermometer with mercury inside, not the digital ones. Shake down the thermometer before you go to bed at night. Stick it under your arm as soon as you wake up and leave it there for ten minutes. Record the temperature before you get out of bed. Follow this procedure for at least six mornings in a row to get the best information. If you are a menstruating woman, your temperature will rise around the time of ovulation because of a hormone surge, so it is best to avoid taking readings mid-cycle. The normal range for resting temperature is 97.8 to 98.2 degrees F. If your temperature is below 97.8 degrees F you have a low-functioning thyroid (hypothyroid). According to the Dr. Broda O. Barnes Foundation, hypothyroid people will exhibit any one of over 100 symptoms, and no two people will have the same symptoms. However, some overt signs of a low-functioning thyroid are: fatigue, constipation, cold hands and feet, dry skin, loss of the outer third of your eyebrow, hyperlaxity of joints (being double-jointed), and backward-facing palms of your hands when you stand.

Some people need prescription thyroid medication to boost their levels of thyroid hormone. Most medical doctors have been trained to prescribe Synthroid, which needs to be split by liver enzymes before it can work in the cell. Mercury and other toxins may inhibit the enzyme from being able to activate the Synthroid. In addition, the receptor sites for the hormones on your cells can get filled up by mercury and other toxic substances preventing thyroid hormone from binding to your cells and stimulating actions such as an increased basal metabolic rate and increased energy production. Whole-gland prescription medications may be helpful; they are called Armour Desiccated Thyroid and Naturthroid. The already activated form of thyroid called Cytomel may be helpful. You will need to work with a trained physician to find the right type and dose of thyroid for you (see Appendix 1).

As we have seen, toxicity is a major cause of this malfunction of thyroid stimulation in your cells. Cleansing will help every cell of your body function at a higher level of performance, making you think, feel, and look better. It makes sense to engage in a quality detoxification program before taking prescription medication. It may be all that your body needs to get you back on track to good health.

How Poor Digestion Affects the Lymphatic System

Let's now consider the job of the lymphatic vessels teamed up with the blood vessels in your villi, which are designed to protect your body from harmful microbes. In response to a pathogen, your lymph vessels release fighters to protect your body from being invaded. If you have a well-balanced mind and body, the immune system releases just the right amount of protector cells and natural killer cells to do the job, but if your system is under stress and overburdened with toxins and a diet that causes hypersensitivity reactions, it will surely overreact. The degree of overreaction depends on the extent of your body's overload. The hyper-response may cause a generalized inflammatory reaction in your GI tract, disturbing your ability to absorb nutrients and initiating an inflammatory cascade that may also affect distant parts of your body. Hence, you can get musculoskeletal pain as a result of a germ. Most people can relate to this problem, having experienced soreness and achiness with a cold or flu. Chronic musculoskeletal pain may be related to a chronic imbalance of good versus bad microbes in your GI tract. Periodic cleansing programs are the perfect remedy for such ills.

When you consume more fat in a meal than your body can effectively metabolize (which most Americans do), the excess is swept into the lymph vessels and circulated until your fat digesters can handle more, or it gets stored in fat cells. The Inuit Eskimos of northern Canada eat the fat of sea mammals and fish whose fat contains toxic residues. Along with the fat, the Inuit consume the toxic products of industrial pollution. Toxins get stored in the fat of all plants and animals so even if you aren't eating whale blubber for dinner, you are being exposed to pollution particles from what you eat. These damaging particles can wreak havoc within your immune system, causing damage to cells and a hyperimmune protective response. But while the toxins in fat may cause a hyperimmune response, the presence of excess fat suppresses the ability of your immune system to respond to germs, leaving you more susceptible to infections, colds, and flus. And even if your lymph is activated to react to the toxins in the fat, it may not have the ability to respond to harmful microorganisms.

If your lymph system is congested, you will usually feel enlarged lymph nodes or glands. A good place to check for enlarged lymph nodes and glands is under your jaw in the area between the corners of your mouth and ear. Press up with your fingers; if these glands are tender, you are probably dealing with an acute infection. If they are swollen and non-tender, it may be chronic. Other areas to check for lymph node congestion are at the crease of your leg in the groin area, in your armpits, and along the muscles in the front of your neck and at the base of your skull. A word of caution: sometimes lymph node enlargement is associated with diseases of the lymphatic system and should be checked by your medical doctor. If you do not have a disease, there are suggestions for clearing lymph congestion in Chapter 11.

Elimination via the Skin

Your largest organ of elimination is your skin. It is designed by nature to excrete bodily wastes through your pores and sweat glands. It is essential to let your body perspire, for the sake of your skin and your whole body. In fact, there are detoxification strategies designed around sweating. Historically, people have taken saunas, sweat lodges, and steam baths to purify their bodies.

Dr. William Rea of Dallas, Texas, developed a "cleansing through sweating" protocol designed around moderate exercise, nutritional supplementation—particularly niacin, one of the B-vitamins—and sweating in a low-temperature sauna. The minimum amount of time needed to initiate the cleansing process is two weeks, but he encourage his patients to continue with the cleansing protocols at home on a regular basis. This type of program has tremendous results, particularly in detoxifying people who have a history of anesthesia or prescribed or recreational drug use.

If you have an overload of toxins in your body, you may notice the result as unpleasant conditions of the skin. One patient had skin problems until she began internal cleansing: "A severe rash on my elbows and forearms that I had for many years is clearing up and is almost gone." The importance of the skin and cleansing protocols is discussed in more detail in Chapter 15.

How the Liver and Kidneys Nourish and Detoxify

The liver and kidneys both filter blood and have the challenging task of distinguishing between unwanted toxins and needed nutrients. The kidneys conserve water and balance electrolytes by reabsorbing the exact amounts required minute by minute and sending the excess out through the urinary tract. This is done via a sophisticated network of electrochemical responses, including the brain, nervous system, and endocrine (hormone-producing) glands. If you have been eating a diet high in refined carbohydrates and sugar, and low or deficient in good fats, your body simply won't have the raw material available to make the hormones it needs.

The liver is a complex organ that both stores nutrients and detoxifies the bloodstream. All blood that leaves the intestines goes through the liver first before it is sent out to the rest of your body. Your liver acts as a shield to ensure that harmful substances absorbed through your gut wall are made safe or stored in a relatively non-active fatty tissue. Taking NSAIDs inhibits the liver's ability to detoxify; the body's safety net is breached, and the floodgates are left open for damaging substances to harm your every cell.

One of the functions of the liver is to *deconjugate,* or break down, hormones. If the liver is damaged by excess fat, toxins, drugs, or alcohol you can end up with too many hormones in your bloodstream. This is a major factor in premenstrual syndrome (PMS). The hormones involved in the menstrual cycle promote water retention and cause bloating even in the brain, which creates some of the emotional tension that women feel during menstruation. An excess of hormones in the bloodstream may also contribute to the increasing incidence of cancer in both men's and women's sex glands because of hormone overstimulation. Women who have a longer exposure to their own estrogen through more frequent menstrual periods and a higher total number of menstrual cycles have a higher incidence of breast, ovary, and uterine cancers.

Look for these signs and symptoms of liver distress:

- acne and other skin disorders
- inability to digest fats, which may show up as nausea or light-colored stools
- constipation or diarrhea
- pain between your shoulder blades, especially on your right side
- pain in your muscles between the neck and shoulder
- headaches, especially ones that begin in the neck/shoulder area and travel up the side of your head around your ear and into your eye
- anger and irritability
- multiple allergies/sensitivities

Blood tests can reveal liver pathology, but there is a simple at-home test you can do to determine if you would benefit from liver cleansing: Lie on your back with your knees bent and your feet flat. Place the fingers of both hands at the edge of your rib cage on the right side on a line directly below your nipple. Inhale deeply and as you exhale press your fingers firmly up under your rib cage in the direction of your head

If this causes pain—especially if it makes you draw your breath in sharply and stop breathing—you should consult a trained health care professional who can guide you in a liver cleansing program. If you have discomfort but not pain, you would be wise to engage in some of the cleansing suggestions recommended in the following chapters and, in addition, take a look at what you can change in your lifestyle to decrease your toxic load.

CHAPTER 3

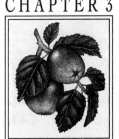

NATURAL ELEMENTS OF A CLEAN BOWEL

Perhaps the most frequently reported bowel problem that people experience is constipation. Constipation is commonly related to a low-fiber diet, which causes fecal matter to become condensed and compressed. Evacuation then becomes infrequent and difficult. There are five major factors to consider when you have sluggish elimination from your bowel. We will investigate each of these five areas briefly:

1. Are you getting enough fiber in your diet?
2. Are you drinking adequate amounts of pure water?
3. Does your diet include high-quality essential fatty acids?
4. Do you pay attention when nature calls?
5. Do you get enough exercise?

In the past decade, the terms "constipated" and "regularity" have been redefined by medical research. A *constipated* system is one in which the transition time of toxic waste matter is slow and the consistency of the stool causes strain. The longer the transit time, the longer the toxic waste matter sits in the bowel, allowing proteins to putrefy, fats to become rancid, and carbohydrates to ferment. The longer your body is exposed to rotting food in your intestines, the greater your risk of developing disease. Even with one bowel movement per day, you still have at least three meals' worth of waste sitting in your colon most of the time.

During evacuation, hard stools place a strain on the colonic muscles and on the lining of the lower portion of your large intestine, rectum, and anus. Straining contributes to the formation of hemorrhoids, varicose veins, hiatal hernia, and a host of other mechanically induced problems. Your system can also become polluted by poisonous gases caused by stagnation in your bowel. These gases can enter your bloodstream, irritating your organs and joints. Alternating constipation and diarrhea or diarrhea alone are also indications of foulness in your intestines. Finally, the much more serious and life-threatening problems of cancer and immune system disorders begin inside a toxic bowel. I will recommend effective strategies for overcoming all of these health challenges throughout *Internal Cleansing*.

Recently, two patients came to my office suffering with serious constipation. One was having, at best, five bowel movements per week. The other said he had eliminated only once every four days since he was a small boy. Perhaps your intestines have a similar rhythm of malfunction, and perhaps your medical doctor—like that of the first patient—has told you that this level of excretion is okay. Her doctor's perspective was that some people just have fewer bowel movements than others. That is true, but what he neglected to tell her is that those who have fewer bowel movements are harboring a breeding ground for disease and death.

After reading this book, you will understand why infrequent bowel movements are dangerous to your health. Once you have learned, please advise others who have slow-moving bowels about the importance of freely flowing waste products in the intestinal tract. Dr. Anthony Bassler, a gastroenterologist, says to his colleagues, "Every physician should realize that the intestinal toxemias are the most important primary and contributing causes of many disorders and diseases of the human body."

Let's take a look at what happens to the shape of your lower intestines when toxic matter has built up on your intestinal walls for years (Figure 3.1). When the colon becomes impacted with dry putrefactive waste, its shape and function are affected in many ways. It will stretch like a balloon in certain areas, or develop diverticula (pouches on the intestinal wall), or fall upon itself (a condition called *prolapsus*). All of these malformations greatly impair your large intestine's ability to function, which in turn places severe strain on your digestive organs and glands.

Frequently, lower back pain, neck and shoulder pain, wrist and hand pain, skin problems, "brain fog," fatigue, sluggishness, and colds and flus are caused by a blocked or slow-moving bowel. Even the common headache can be attributed to bowel dysfunction. Neurological problems are made worse by toxicity. A male patient in his fifties who has an abnormal walk due to a disc problem in his neck found that he walked better and felt more balanced after doing an internal cleansing program designed for his particular needs.

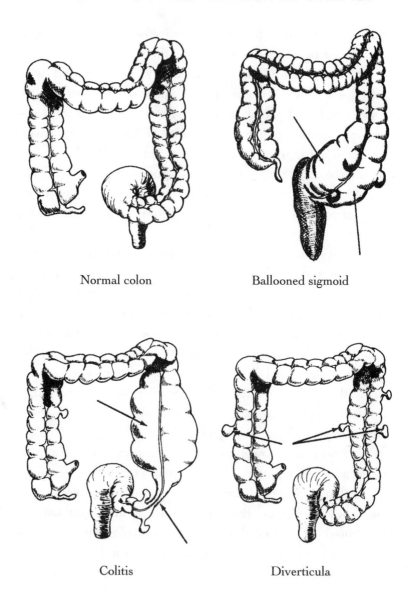

Normal colon   Ballooned sigmoid

Colitis   Diverticula

Figure 3.1   Colon Dysfunctions.

Reprinted, by permission, from *Tissue Cleansing Through Bowel Management* by Dr. Bernard Jensen.

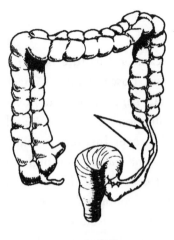

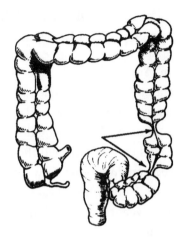

Spasm   Stricture

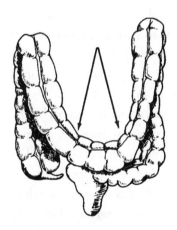

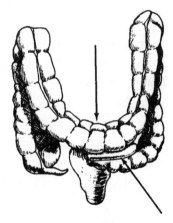

Prolapsus   Prolapsus with pressure
                                 on lower organs

Figure 3.1   (continued)

THE ROLE OF FIBER IN INTESTINAL HEALTH

In August of 1984, the National Cancer Institute issued a statement called "Dietary Fiber and Lower Colon Cancer Risk," which states: "Research data suggesting that fiber-containing foods provide some protection against colon and rectal cancer have led the National Cancer Institute to make recommendations now that Americans eat a diet high in fiber from whole grain breads and cereals and fresh fruits and vegetables. If followed, these recommendations may reduce individual risk of these cancers." The statement goes on to affirm that "basic relationships between intake of fiber-containing foods and human cancer are now firmly established in the scientific literature."

On average, Americans get only about 15 grams, half the fiber necessary, every day. A shocking 25 percent of Americans get only five to seven grams per day or less. No wonder there are so many digestive problems in our population, or that $700 million worth of laxatives is sold every year. No wonder so many of us suffer with hemorrhoids, appendicitis, ulcerative colitis, diverticular disease, adenomatous polyps (considered to be early markers of colon cancer development), colon cancer, and heart disease.

Denis P. Burkitt, M.D., a physician who worked extensively with native peoples in Africa, wrote about the link between low-fiber diets and increased risk of modernization diseases in his landmark December 1969 article in *The Lancet*, a peer-reviewed medical journal. He noted that the conditions listed above were "exceedingly rare" in rural Africa. However, as their diets became more Western

(SAD) with decreased amounts of fiber, increased amounts of refined carbohydrates, in particular white flour products, and increased amounts of fat, the rural Africans experienced a rise in the incidence of these troubling conditions and life-threatening diseases.

Because a lack of fiber causes slower movement of feces through your bowel, it allows carcinogenic substances to be in contact with your intestinal wall longer. This could lead to possible formation of colon cancer—the third leading cause of cancer deaths in the United States (see Figure 3.2 for the beneficial properties of fiber).

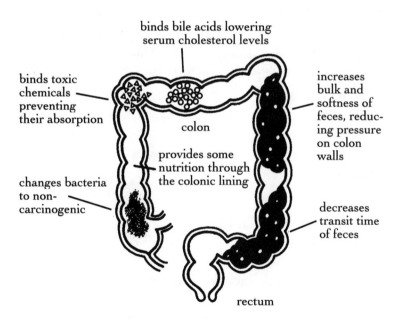

Figure 3.2   The Protective Properties of Fiber

Fiber and Lignins

Fiber also provides nutrition to your bowel flora—the friendly microorganisms in your intestines that work to promote your health. If these bacteria are fed well with certain types of plant fibers they reproduce in greater numbers and produce a substance called *mammalian lignan,* which increases your resistance to infectious agents and cancer. Plant fibers are the preferred source of food for your friendly bacteria. They will convert to taking in nutrients from the bowel only during times of fasting or starvation.

The fiber in flaxseed generates one hundred times more lignans than any other fiber source. (Flaxseed is one of the best sources of essential fatty acids; see "Essential Fatty Acids" later in this chapter.) Breast cancer patients, and others at high risk for colon and breast cancer, excrete far fewer lignans than healthy people. This implies that they have fewer lignins present in their bowel than do people without these types of cancers. To decrease your risk of getting breast or colon cancer, include fresh ground flaxseed—also called flax meal—in your diet on a regular basis.

For more information on dietary fiber, please see Chapter 7.

THE ROLE OF WATER IN INTESTINAL HEALTH

If you do not drink enough water, your body will dry out and it will be difficult to have a bowel movement. It is impossible to overstate the importance of pure water. Your body is mostly water—fifty to seventy-five percent. You will absorb some water through your skin by soaking in a bathtub or by swimming, but your main source is, of course, drinking water. You need to drink water because every day you lose water through sweat, urine, and breath.

How many glasses of water do you drink each day? Many people are so out of touch with sufficient water consumption that they don't even know they are thirsty; they have suppressed their internal message to rehydrate by making the busywork of life a priority over taking care of their basic health needs. Generally, six to eight glasses (eight ounces per glass) of water per day is recommended for the average adult. However, for detoxification purposes you will need more water (see Chapter 13 for specific quantities).

The quality of your health is directly related to the quality of your drinking water (see Chapter 6 to learn about water quality standards). Most importantly, drink pure water on a daily basis for your best health. (For further discussions on water consumption, the environment, and filtration, see Chapters 5 and 6.)

ESSENTIAL FATTY ACIDS

Essential fatty acids (EFAs) play a role in hormone and immune system function, both of which are critical to bowel health. They provide the raw materials from which your body produces hormones. EFAs also provide for the smooth functioning of your immune system for the free flow of blood through your arteries and veins, forming sheaths around your nerves to protect the integrity of information transmission along your nerves. Your hormones, immune system, vascular system (arteries and veins), and nervous system all coordinate to ensure a healthy bowel. Hormones activate movement in your intestinal muscles to aid digestion and elimination. Your immune system protects the rest of your body from invasion by toxic substances and pathogenic microorganisms that can otherwise pass from your bowel into your body. Your immune system also regulates the amount of inflammation in your intestines. Your arteries and veins supply nourishment to the cells that line your intestines and take away toxic metabolites. Your nerves command the function of every cell in your body, including your intestines, and carry information on the status of your bowel back to your brain so it knows what to do to regulate normal function. (See Appendix 3 for more information on EFAs.)

As their name implies, EFAs are essential to human health. According to Edward Siguel, M.D., in his book *Essential Fatty Acids in Health and Disease*, "Without essential fats, cells do not work, organs die prematurely, brain function deteriorates." In nutritional literature, nutrients are called "essential" because your body cannot make them; you must get them from your diet or from nutritional supplements.

When I review a list of all of the food, condiments, and beverages my patients have consumed for a week, I find that 100 percent of the time they are either deficient or totally lacking in EFAs. Experts agree that a diet deficient in EFAs is hazardous to your health. Your body is made up of 100 trillion cells, and every cell needs EFAs to make its cell wall and to burn for energy. The gray matter in the human brain is fifty percent EFAs. Infants and young children are especially vulnerable to EFA deficiency states because their brains and bodies are developing and adding mass. If EFAs are not available from their mothers' milk or in their diet, normal brain, nervous system, immune system, and heart development may not occur.

The recommended quantity of EFA supplementation is one teaspoon of flaxseed oil per day for each thirty-five pounds of body weight. As indicated by the following chart, a person weighing between 105 and 139 pounds would need to consume up to four teaspoons of flaxseed oil per day to achieve and maintain optimal health (three teaspoons equal one tablespoon).

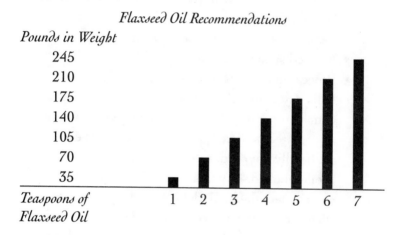

Flaxseed Oil Recommendations

Pounds in Weight

Teaspoons of Flaxseed Oil

Two important classes of EFAs are *omega-3* and *omega-6*. Omega-3 EFAs can be found in reliable quantities in flaxseed oil and fresh water fish. They can be found in small amounts in pumpkin seeds and walnuts. It is important to take in these nutrients in a healthy balance. Unfortunately, the type of diet we eat today supplies only one-eighth of the omega-3 content of the traditional hunter/gatherer diet, which helped us evolve into beings with a large brain-to-body ratio. To further complicate your omega-3 deficiency, modern food processing and lifestyles create *antinutrients* that call for even higher doses of omega-3 EFAs to balance their toxic effects. These antinutrients include:

- Saturated fat in the form of animal fats from meat, eggs, full-fat dairy products, and the skin of poultry.
- Altered fats called *trans fatty acids* in margarine and other hydrogenated, partially hydrogenated, and fractionated vegetable oils commonly found in chips, crackers, salad dressings, icings, candy bars, and baked goods (health-food-store candy is frequently made with partially fractionated palm kernel oil—an especially damaging trans fat).
- Peanut butter, peanuts, and peanut oil.
- Refined sugar and flour.
- Processed foods (Dr. Donald Rudin and Clara Felix say that, before supermarket food reaches your plate, it may have been: acidified, antibiotically treated, antioxidated, artificially colored, artificially flavored, artificially supplemented, broiled/boiled, bromated, chemically enriched, chlorinated, defatted, defibered, dehydrated, emulsified, fried, hybridized, hydrogenated, marbled, nitrated, phosphated, salted, and/or sugared; see Appendix 3 for information on their books).
- Caffeine, alcohol, and cigarettes.
- Recreational, prescription, and over-the-counter drugs.

For better health, minimize saturated animal fat in your diet and balance what you do eat with sources of omega-3 EFAs. If you have arthritis or other inflammatory conditions, you may see improvements if you eliminated the saturated animal fat altogether. Throw out any trans fatty acids and minimize eating out because restaurant food is loaded with trans fats. Peanut butter should not be eaten by anyone with an inflammatory condition because it promotes pain and swelling. Refined sugar and flour are not good for you, but if you do eat them, make up for it by eating more fruits and vegetables. Processed food and cigarettes only do harm. Caffeine and alcohol in small amounts are okay if you insist on using them. As for drugs of all sorts, seek alternatives first and use only as a final option.

Our ancestors got their omega-3 EFAs from fish, shellfish, and mollusks; land and water plants; nuts and seeds; and wild game. Examine your own diet to see how much high-quality food of this nature you eat on a daily basis. Omega-6 EFAs come from warm weather oils such as safflower, canola, and soybeans and in the seeds and oils of sesame, sunflower, walnut, and pumpkin. They are essential, but more readily available in the American diet, though some may need to supplement with these oils as well. In order for the omega-3 fatty acids to perform their vital functions, other essential nutrients (proteins, vitamins, and minerals) must be present in your diet in adequate amounts. And, on the other side of the fat equation, substances antagonistic to EFAs must be eliminated or dramatically reduced. (See Appendix 3 for more information on this vital health issue.)

Americans have been concerned about reducing the quantity of fats and oils they consume. Despite their efforts, however, thirty percent more Americans are obese now than in 1970. How can that be? Many in the nutritional field attribute this trend at least partially to the reduction or elimination of EFAs from our diets. Udo Erasmus, in *Fats That Heal, Fats That Kill*, states, "[EFAs] stimulate metabolism, increase metabolic rate and oxidation, and speed up the rate at which our bodies burn fats and glucose when they get more than twelve to fifteen percent of total calories as EFAs.

In these quantities (upwards of three tablespoons per day), EFAs burn off excess fat and help a person to lose weight and stay slim." In *The Facts About Fats*, John Finnegan describes the experience of people who added EFAs to their daily diet: "Many of my friends and clients report that, after adding in one to two tablespoons a day of flaxseed oil to their diets, they have lost their cravings for fatty foods and have experienced continued weight loss, increased energy, and a sense of dietary satisfaction."

This happy occurrence is brought to us by EFAs' regulation of *brown fat*, a metabolically active form of fat that maintains body temperature by burning calories. Brown fat is concentrated around the spine and organs.

TRANS FATTY ACIDS

A discussion of trans fatty acids (TFAs) is warranted here. TFAs cause damage to your cells. They interfere with and inhibit all of the functions of omega-3 EFAs. TFAs dramatically increase the amount of toxins your body must deal with, inhibiting cleansing and destroying health (see Figure 3.3).

cis fatty acid	*trans* fatty acid
The H's are on the same side of the double bond, forcing the molecule to assume horseshoe shape.	The H's are on opposite sides of the double bond, forcing the molecule into an extended position.

Figure 3.3   Cis vs. *Trans* Fatty Acid Configuration

TFAs are produced by the current food processing techniques. In order to increase shelf life and increase the marketability of oil, modern food technology experts violated the healthy chemical configuration of vegetable oils. In his book, *The Facts About Fats*, John Finnegan notes, "The effects of poorly processed oils are a major factor in heart disease, cancer and most modern diseases that have affected hundreds of millions of people all over the world."

Nature provides us with vegetable oils in a chemical form called the cis configuration. The form provided to us in nature is biologically active, meaning that your body can break it down into its tiny constituents and make it into the stuff of you. The *trans* form made by man is not biologically active, meaning that you have been unknowingly cheating your body of needed nutrition when you eat a trans fat.

The most common source of these trans fats is margarine. The public has been led to believe that margarine will protect them from developing heart disease. Unfortunately, the reverse is true. Eating margarine and other forms of trans fats will increase your risk of death by heart disease. Researchers believe this happens because the altered oil damages your cells and robs them of the nutrients needed to protect you from chronic degenerative diseases. Altered oils and the deficiency of EFAs have been implicated not only in the causation of heart disease but also in such health conditions as:

1. Inflammatory conditions such as colitis, diverticulitis, sinusitis, gingivitis, gastritis, and arthritis
2. Immune system dysfunction
3. Hormone regulation problems including PMS, menstrual cramps, infertility, impotence, vaginal dryness, and prostate enlargement

4. Allergic disorders
5. Chorn's Disease
6. Retinal blindness
7. Diabetes
8. Skin disorders such as acne, eczema, psoriasis, seborrheic dermatitis, dandruff, dry, cracked and scaling skin, sun sensitivity, sudden hair loss in defined patches and rough, prickly skin on the upper arms, elbows, thighs and buttocks are aggravated by trans fats
9. Childhood problems such as Sudden Infant Death Syndrome (SIDS), Attention Deficit Disorder (ADD), autism, and dental problems
10. Manic depressive disorder, anxiety, schizophrenia, and agoraphobia
11. Aging: wrinkles, age spots, graying hair, glaucoma

In order to get the highest quality oils, buy those that are organic and have been processed in the absence of light and air with presses of a size that you can get your arms around. Refer to the list of resources in Appendix 1 of this book for a listing of these suppliers.

To enjoy the benefits of EFAs, build your diet around plenty of omega-3 and omega-6 EFAs. Food sources of these essential healing oils are: cold-water fish, including salmon, mackerel, cod, and halibut; walnuts, flaxseed, and sesame, sunflower, and pumpkin seeds or their oils; lentils; and leafy green vegetables.

Flaxseed oil, a highly nutritious oil rich in EFAs, is usually manufactured and distributed in opaque plastic containers. Unfortunately, it is difficult to find fresh, high-quality oils in the United States. When you do find them, they are more expensive than other oils—approximately $30 more per person per year—but considering the damage that improperly produced oil can cause, it is worth the investment (see Appendix 1 for recommended sources).

WHEN NATURE CALLS, RESPOND

Finally, paying attention "when nature calls" is essential to smoothly functioning bowels. Physiologically, human beings operate on a stimulus/response basis in regard to bodily functions. If you repeatedly ignore the urge to eliminate, you interfere with your body's ability to respond appropriately. Sooner or later, your body won't be able to function without artificial stimulation from medication, herbs, or water therapies such as enemas and colonics.

It is best to plan for proper elimination if you have a challenge in this area. Leave enough time in the morning after eating to allow the oral/anal reflex to work. When you chew food, you stimulate the inside of your mouth and a cascade of electrical and chemical events fires off, activating *peristalsis* within your gastrointestinal (GI) tract. Peristalsis is the muscular contraction that propels food down your digestive canal and feces out of your body. To respect your body's natural rhythms and to allow for easy elimination, it is helpful to be near a bathroom within an hour of eating.

EXERCISE THE WASTE OUT OF YOUR BODY

If you want to have healthy, smoothly functioning bowels, it is important to engage in a regular exercise program, or at least to step up your activity level. All of the muscles in your body respond favorably to appropriate exercise, including the smooth muscle of your intestinal tract. The benefits of exercise have also been proven scientifically. A study involving people 65 and over showed that the group that exercised on a regular basis had more frequent and less difficult bowel movements than the group that did not.

In the 1970s before I knew about internal cleansing and all the steps you can take to support a healthy intestinal tract, my favorite remedy for constipation was to eat a raw carrot and go for a walk. That remedy was double-strength in that it included both the fiber and the exercise that stimulate bowel motility. Often one remedy alone will not work, but when combined with others, the force for healing multiplies. For more information about exercise, see Chapter 15.

PART II:

TOXINS IN OUR
FOOD AND
ENVIRONMENT

CHAPTER 4

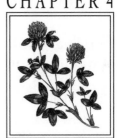

TOXINS IN FOOD

THE IMPACT OF DIET ON TOXIC BUILDUP IN THE BODY

The Western diet has changed more in the last two centuries than at any previous time in human history. The changes have provided many conveniences, but they have also created new health threats. Chronic degenerative diseases build slowly and insidiously over a period of years until they gradually disrupt some part of your body. The most common killers are cardiovascular disease (disease of the heart and blood circulation system), cancers in the body, gastrointestinal diseases or disorders, arthritis, emphysema and other lung diseases, diabetes, and other endocrine system disorders. Medical science has proven that changes in our diet and lifestyle play an enormous role in the development of these diseases. Many of these diseases can be prevented by making informed changes in what you eat, what you think, how you move, and even in how you relate to your fellow human beings.

WHAT'S WRONG WITH THE AMERICAN DIET?

Since industrialization began over two hundred years ago, the Western diet has become increasingly rich in meats, poultry, fish, saturated fats, refined foods, salt, and sugar. Our over-generous intake of animal fats has burdened our cardiovascular systems with cholesterol, our kidneys with protein, and our livers with animal hormones, alcohol, and drugs. Processed foods, which account for *more than half* of Americans' food intake, are loaded with salts, sugars, preservatives, and artificial, chemically altered ingredients. Every year, Americans spend more money on alcohol than our government does on the defense budget. We drink more soft drinks and coffee than ever before.

This change in diet is due to a new affluence in industrialized countries, to the availability of a wide variety of foods because of refrigeration and shipping, and to the overstimulation of our appetite centers by advertising campaigns of the food industry. The net result of these dietary changes since the beginning of this century has been a thirty-two-percent increase in fat consumption, a fifty-percent increase in consumption of sugar and other sweeteners, and a forty-three-percent increase in consumption of carbohydrates. Increased consumption of fat (especially trans fats, which constitute up to twenty percent of the American diet) and refined carbohydrates leads to increased risk of heart disease, cancer, and diabetes, to name a few diseases that have escalated with the modernization of the Western World.

Junk Food

Since the beginning of the twentieth century, the modern diet has become increasingly worse. Dr. Michael T. Murray, a naturopathic physician, provides the following statistics on the startling amount of junk food the average Americans consume annually:

   100 pounds of refined sugar
   55 pounds of fats and oils
   300 cans of soda pop
   200 sticks of gum
   18 pounds of candies
   5 pounds of potato chips
   63 dozen donuts
   20 gallons of ice cream

Our national annual total for cola consumption is 100 billion ounces, and we spend $50 million on Twinkies. The food industry spends $8 billion annually on advertising these products. Over thirty percent of Americans smoke cigarettes, and more than seven percent are active alcoholics. On average, produce is shipped 1,800 miles before it reaches your table. In order to remain intact during shipping, the produce must be picked before it is fully ripe, and it sits in warehouses, in trucks, and on the grocery store shelves for days before you buy it. This means that the nutritive value is underdeveloped and depleted before the fruit or vegetable becomes food for your body.

Sugar

The average American consumes a shocking 100 pounds of sugar per year, which translates to approximately one-third pound per day. Excess intake of sugar has been found to contribute to a wide variety of health problems, from tooth decay to heart disease, diabetes, hypoglycemia, obesity, and vaginal infections. Right from the start, babies' taste buds are perverted by the addition of simple sugars to baby formulas. I have seen mothers fill up bottles for their infants with artificially colored orange soda, and grandmothers put sugar in the water they serve to their grandchildren, beginning a lifetime addiction to sugar. In this chapter, you will learn why feeding your infant sugar sets them up to struggle with weight problems for the rest of their lives.

Salt

On average, Americans consume a whopping eight pounds of salt per year. Have you ever read the ingredient label on a container of commercial table salt? It lists salt, sodium silicoaluminate, dextrose, potassium iodide, and sodium bicarbonate. What are all of these things doing in our salt? The addition of sodium silicoaluminate allows salt manufacturers to say that their salt is free-flowing. Putting some rice grains in your salt shaker can accomplish the same result without adding aluminum to your diet. Aluminum has been found in high concentrations in the brains of people with Alzheimer's disease. Dextrose (sugar) makes the salt taste sweet. Potassium iodide was added to salt after people in the Midwest, deprived of sources of ocean fish, developed goiter (enlargement of the thyroid gland). Sodium bicarbonate is an alkalizing agent, added to neutralize the acidity caused by the addition of the sweetness of the dextrose. Salt comes from two places: the sea, and dried up ocean beds in the desert. If you want to have a purer form of salt, buy sea salt from your health food store or rock salt from the supermarket. Neither of these forms of salt has the additives of commercial table salt. However, they may be without the trace minerals you should be getting from natural salt sources. Look for *unre-*

fined sea salt, or you may end up with a product containing only sodium chloride.

Fats

The daily intake of calories from fat has more than tripled in the past two centuries, and the increase is mainly in the form of animal fat. Scientific data indicate that a diet rich in animal fat is strongly related to a high risk of heart disease and cancers of the colon, breast, and uterus. Heart disease is the leading cause of death in both Britain and America today, killing one out of every three people. Since it is difficult to digest large amounts of fat, this excess may also lead to constipation, diarrhea, liver and gall bladder problems, menstrual and premenstrual difficulties, and skin disorders.

Low Fiber Intake

As you read in Chapter 3, fiber is an important element of good bowel health. Fiber also plays an important preventive role for many degenerative diseases, primarily heart disease, diabetes, and colon and hormone-related cancers. According to statistics, our daily intake of fiber is greatly reduced because of the consumption of refined and processed foods. Fresh fruits and vegetables and whole grains, as opposed to refined rice or flour products, must be included in your daily diet to achieve a sufficient fiber supply for health and well-being. Some of you will not manage to ingest in your diet the thirty to sixty grams of fiber per day that is necessary for optimal health, so in Chapter 7, I will discuss fiber supplements you can take to enhance your daily fiber supply.

Overeating

With the change in diet and the lack of exercise in our daily schedules, it is easy to gain ten to twenty pounds of excess weight. Weight gain may negatively impact your level of energy and self-esteem. It takes more energy to move more weight around and if you are unhappy with your weight you carry the additional psychological burden of disapproving of your body and yourself for not managing your weight better. Both of these factors contribute to depleting your energy reserves. As was discussed in Chapter 1, negative self-talk leads to increased toxicity. Most likely the quality of the food and/or the proportion of protein, carbohydrate, and fat are not optimal resulting in an increased toxic load. Experts in cardiovascular disease estimate that at least one-fourth of all heart disease problems can be attributed to overeating, which forces the heart and lungs to work harder than is healthy for them.

Body Composition Analysis with skin calipers, bio-impedance analysis, or immersion can measure the percentage of your weight that comes from fat, lean tissue such as muscle, bone and tendons, and water. Skin calipers measure body composition by measuring the depth of skin folds with a pinching device in places where fat usually accumulates (under the upper arm, the waist, etc.). Bio-impedance analysis is a state of the art tool that measures reactance and resistance to an extremely light electrical current that runs from two electrodes placed on one hand and foot on the same side of your body. The measures are then entered into a computer that calculates percentages. Immersion in water is the last technique. After you are covered with grease and dressed in a bathing suit, you are immersed in a tub of water up to your neck. With this method, buoyancy and water displacement are the measures used to calculate body composition.

Body Composition Analysis is very helpful in guiding you through a cleansing program to ensure that you are not losing your vital lean tissue. Obesity is considered to be a measure of body fat equal to or greater than thirty percent of your total body weight. Obesity is the leading cause of high blood pressure, which in turn causes kidney damage, heart disease, and stroke. Hypertension is twice as common among overweight people as among lean people. Fat people have approximately four times the risk of developing diabetes, and an increased risk of varicose veins, gout, respiratory diseases, gastrointestinal disorders, gall bladder and liver diseases, and arthritis. These conditions are all "itises" that respond favorably to internal cleansing.

One of the most significant signs of risk for heart disease and diabetes is a waist to hip ratio that is greater than 0.95 for women and 0.75 for men. You can determine your ratio by measuring your waist (the smallest measurement between the bottom of your rib cage and above your naval) and your hips (the largest measurement around the widest part of your buttocks and upper thighs). Then divide your waist measurement by your hip measurement. For example, if you are a woman with a waist measurement of 28 and a hip measurement of 38, your ratio is 28 ÷ 38 = 0.74, well within the limits of safety. If your ratio is higher than the upper limit, it does not necessarily mean that you will manifest either disease, especially if you use your new found knowledge to take action steps to improve your health.

In order to understand weight gain, we have to consider the nutritional value of food. The fundamental reason all creatures eat is to satisfy their nutritional requirements for living. Only human beings have developed food into a culinary art. When you eat sugar, alcohol, candy, and other refined carbohydrates (pasta, sourdough or white bread, rolls, cookies, cakes, and pastries) you drive up your need to eat more food, yet you feel satisfied only briefly because you are consuming "empty calories." Whenever you ingest a food or beverage other than pure water, you engage the metabolic (digestive) machinery in your body. The process of digestion requires energy and uses up key nutrients that are stored for this purpose. Refined foods do not contain the nutrients you need for their digestion, so you end up depleting your body's warehouse of stored nutrients. Because your basic needs are not met, you continue to be hungry, so you eat more than your body, mind, and heart need to thrive.

Caffeine

Twenty to thirty percent of American adults consume more than 500 milligrams of caffeine per day—twice the amount doctors consider a large "drug dose." An eight-ounce cup of coffee contains approximately 136 milligrams of caffeine. That means it takes four cups of coffee to total 544 milligrams of caffeine. Coffee, tea, cola beverages, and chocolate in all of its forms are the major sources of this caffeine consumption. Caffeine is also found in over-the-counter and prescription drugs. Studies performed in the past ten years indicate that caffeine users have a 100 percent greater than average risk of heart attack.

There are several reasons to quit drinking coffee. Coffee is a narcotic beverage. The caffeine in your coffee belongs in the same alkaloid group of chemicals as morphine, cocaine, and strychnine. Drinking decaffeinated coffee is probably no better than drinking "hi-test" because of the large concentration of trichloroethylene (TCE), a potent liver carcinogen. Furthermore, growers use more pesticides on this crop than on any other. Some of the pesticides used on coffee plants over the past twenty years are Aldrin, Dieldrin, Chlordane, and Heptachlor. As if the toxic ingredients were not enough, the roasting process that brings out the aroma turns the oils in coffee into dangerous trans fats (discussed in the EFA section of Chapter 3). Nitrosamines, a naturally occurring poison in coffee, are the same carcinogens that we avoid in bacon and other cured meats.

Ingesting caffeine places stress on your heart. Many people feel their heart race when they take their daily dose of caffeine. Because it drives your nervous system into a state of sympathetic alert — the state you attain when a wild animal is chasing you and you are running for your life — you become depleted in B-vitamins, especially B_1 or thiamin (symptoms of vitamin B_1 deficiency include fatigue, nervousness, general malaise, general aches and pains, and headaches). Some people say they feel little of this "buzz" when they drink coffee. That is cause for real concern. If your adrenals do not react to the stimulation of caffeine, it could mean that you are headed for a physical breakdown due to adrenal exhaustion.

When you get into a state of sympathetic alert, your digestive system turns off because your blood is now sent preferentially to your muscles, lungs, and heart. If you have any food in your digestive tract, it is subject to fermentation, putrefaction, and becoming rancid from sitting too long in an intestinal tract that is shut down. Instead of being nourished by your food you will become poisoned by the rotting products of incomplete digestion.

Coffee also interferes with your blood sugar metabolism. By stimulating a sympathetic response, it drives your blood sugar levels up and jolts your pancreas into action, flooding your system with insulin to normalize blood sugar levels. This puts your energy on a roller coaster ride all day long. People on this ride usually go from one caffeine high to the next, wearing out their glands and organs.

Because coffee is highly acidic, drinking it can lead to a deficiency of healthy bacteria in your intestines and make you subject to a host of health problems, including acne, constipation, diarrhea, recurring colds and flu, colitis, irritable bowel syndrome, and fibromyalgia.

If you still feel that you can't live without the buzz of coffee, try some green tea instead. Japanese green tea is high in a substance called *catechin*. This flavonoid complex increases human resistance to certain types of cancers. You could also try jasmine tea or Earl Grey tea, both of which have lovely aromas.

Alcohol

When you drink an alcoholic beverage, it becomes a digestive priority and must be fully metabolized before anything else can be digested. The food you eat along with the alcohol you drink sits in your intestines waiting for its turn like a plane delayed on the runway. Depending on your ethnic background, your food may have a long wait. Native Americans, people of Irish descent, and Asians have a distinct disadvantage in relation to alcohol because of a genetic paucity of the enzyme *alcohol dehydrogenase*, which breaks down and neutralizes alcohol.

Alcohol consumption places a strain on the normal functions of your body. Alcohol disrupts our cells' ability to take in and use nutrients from food. It interferes with the absorption of numerous amino acids and increases the loss of certain vitamins in the urine, including pyridoxine and pantothenic acid (B-complex factors). Drinking denies us the full benefit of what we eat. Heavy drinkers take in so many calories from alcohol that they tend to eat smaller quantities of nutritious food. To summarize, alcohol robs your body of nutrients essential for life.

Of course, we must remember the Taoist proverb, "Even moderation in moderation." There's nothing wrong with having an occasional drink unless it makes you sick or drives you into an alcoholic lifestyle from which you are in recovery.

TOXINS IN FOOD

Food, which is meant to nourish us, has become a significant source of internal pollution, some by design and some by carelessness. Some 2,800 additives are intentionally added to what we eat. (For more on food processing, see page 44.) According to the book *Well Body, Well Earth,* the average American consumes about fourteen pounds of additives a year. As many as 10,000 more additives find their way into food indirectly as it is grown, processed, packaged, and stored. These chemicals include hormones and antibiotics fed to animals, pesticides used on plants and crops, residues from substances used to clean equipment, molecules from plastic wrap, and lead from soldered cans. The Food and Drug Administration does not require that these chemicals be listed on labels.

Chemically Altered Foods

Dr. George Goodheart, a chiropractor and founder of Applied Kinesiology, believes that males are being nutritionally castrated by the presence of trans fats, such as margarine, in our diets. These trans fats are also found in chips, crackers, salad dressings, candies, cake frosting, and other processed foods and are called partially hydrogenated, hydrogenated, or fractionated on the product label. Food companies take a perfectly good food—a polyunsaturated vegetable oil—and add hydrogen atoms to the double bonds in the long carbon chain attached to the hydroxyl portion of the fat. This alteration makes the oil a more chemically stable compound with a longer shelf life. Unfortunately, the longer shelf life is dangerous to human life.

Plastics in Food

In 1988, Drs. Ana Soto and Carlos Sonnenschein of Tufts University made an unexpected discovery while doing cancer research: "Phantom estrogen" coming from the plastic tubes in which they cultured their samples was causing experimental breast-cancer cell colonies to multiply alarmingly. Eventually the researchers learned that the estrogenic substance was *p-nonylphenol,* one of the synthetic chemicals that manufacturers add to polystyrene and polyvinyl chloride (PVC) to make them more stable and less breakable. (P-nonylphenol is also used to synthesize nonoxynol-9 in birth control products such as contraceptive creams, foams, jellies, inserts, films, and condoms.)

Meanwhile, a Stanford University School of Medicine research team found another estrogenic mimic, *bisphenol-A,* in lab flasks and in such consumer products as giant bottled-drinking-water jugs. At the University of Granada, researchers Fatima and Nicolas Olea found bisphenol-A in the plastic coatings that manufacturers use to line metal cans. They further found an astonishingly high concentration of this estrogen mimic in such canned foods as corn, artichokes, and peas. In some instances the cans contained as much as 85 parts per billion bisphenol-A, 27 times the dose that the Stanford team found made breast cancer cells proliferate. The plastic linings are used to avoid possible contamination from tin and lead solder and to protect food from developing a metallic taste; they are found in eighty-five percent of food cans in the United States and forty percent in Spain.

Non-stick cookware is another source of unexpected plastic exposure. The non-stick coating wears away one fleck at a time into your food. For the double whammy toxic effect, your food comes more and more in contact with the aluminum surface underneath as the plastic surface erodes.

Here are some positive steps you can take to minimize the level of plastics in your food:

1. Avoid microwaving food in plastic containers or with microwave plastic wrap. Reheat your food in ceramic or glass containers.
2. Avoid allowing plastic juice and water containers to overheat (keep them out of hot cars and sunlight). If the liquid becomes heated, throw it out. Or else buy juice and water in glass jars and bottles.
3. Avoid eating food from cans. Instead, buy those staples frozen, dried, or in glass jars.

4. Buy food fresh or in glass containers.
5. Throw away your non-stick cookware. Cook your food in steel, glass, ceramic, or cast-iron cookware. Ask about the glaze on ceramics — some contain toxic metals such as lead.
6. Avoid using contraceptive products that contain nonoxynol-9. Seek alternatives.

Bovine Somatotropic Hormone

Since 1994, most cow's milk sold in stores contains bovine somatotropic hormone (BSH). BSH is a synthetic hormone designed to increase a cow's milk production. Cows treated with BSH have a higher incidence of mastitis (a breast infection) and possibly cancers. This hormone passes from the cow's milk into us and our children. The U.S. government does not require labeling of milk and milk products that carry this dangerous hormone. Dairies that do not use BSH may have a statement on their cartons that they never give their cows antibiotics or hormones. Cheeses imported from Europe do not contain BSH. To protect your health, ask your grocer or health food store manager to carry milk and milk products that do not contain this hormone. Or, better yet, drink goat's milk, or get the nutrients you normally derive from milk — primarily protein and calcium — from other food sources.

READ INGREDIENT LABELS

Exercise caution when eating processed food. Read labels carefully, especially the lists of food ingredients and added chemicals. Ask an educated clerk in the store if the list of additives includes helpful vitamin supplements with chemical names that make them sound like toxic additives. Your health care practitioner may also be able to advise you in this regard.

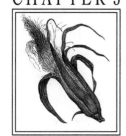

CHAPTER 5

HOUSEHOLD AND OTHER PERSONAL TOXINS

MINIMIZING RISKS INSIDE THE HOME

There is a phenomenon known as "outgassing" of toxic vapors from materials found in the home and office: formaldehyde from particle board furniture, volatile organic compounds (VOCs) from stains and varnishes on wood items and paint on the walls, resins from adhesives that hold furniture and built-in units together, and numerous compounds from plastic household and office items, cleaning products, synthetic carpets, drapes, and upholstery. There are also natural vapors from wood furniture and the furnace, gas range, or woodstove.

Ways to "Clear the Air"

A brochure from the Florida Foliage Association recommends placing approximately 15 plants in an 1,800-square-foot house to combat indoor air pollution. Five plants are listed in their brochure as especially helpful:

- Chinese Evergreen (*Aglaonema 'Silver Queen'*)
- Spider Plant (*Chlorophytum comosum 'Vittatum'*)
- Peace Lily (*Spathiphyllum species*)
- Golden Pothos (*Epipremnum aureum*)
- Weeping Fig (*Ficus benjamina*)

Indoor plants are particularly effective in filtering three chemicals from the air that are responsible for many health problems: benzene, formaldehyde, and trichloroethylene.

Benzene is a common solvent and is present in gasoline, inks, oils, paints, plastic, rubber, detergents, pharmaceuticals, and dyes. It causes symptoms such as: headaches, loss of appetite, drowsiness, nervousness, psychological disturbances, and diseases of the blood system including anemia and bone marrow disease. Evidence also links benzene to cancer, leukemia, liver and kidney damage, paralysis, and unconsciousness.

I have learned that Boston ferns are happy to soak up formaldehyde that out-gasses from particle board and pressed wood furniture and foam insulation in your home or office. Consumer paper products, including grocery bags, waxed paper, facial tissue, and paper towels, are also treated with formaldehyde resins. Formaldehyde irritates the mucous membranes of your eyes and upper respiratory system. Recent research also suggests that it may cause a rare form of throat cancer in long term occupants of mobile homes.

Trichloroethylene (TCE) is used in metal degreasers, dry cleaning agents, inks, paints, lacquers, varnishes, and adhesives. The National Cancer Institute (NCI) considers TCE a potent liver carcinogen. I was informed by one of my patients that if you have 17 spider plants in your home, then your air will be clean. Try what she does: systematically cultivate the "baby spiders" from the first plant in order to reach the recommended quota.

As a part of the photosynthesis process, plants take in carbon dioxide along with airborne toxins and turn them into oxygen for us to breathe. Plants also help clean the air of auto and industrial exhaust, thereby making our world a healthier place for all of us to live. These are only a few reasons why it is so very important for us to protect the plant population on our planet.

You might consider purchasing an air cleaner for your home. They come in a variety of styles; some produce ozone to kill mold, some produce negative ions to precipitate particulate pollutants, and some move air through a carbon filter (to remove gasses) or a HEPA (high-efficiency particulate accumulator) filter. Combination air filters with a charcoal filter and a central HEPA filter are probably the most useful. In my home, I use the combination filter and an ozone generator. In my office, we use a combination filter when necessary (such as when mold or pollution levels are high or when I start to get a headache or "brain fog"). Check *Consumer Reports* for valuable information on this topic.

Household Cleaning Products: Safer Alternatives

You can get rid of all of the toxic cleaners lurking under your sinks and clean an entire house with just a few simple solutions of baking soda, white vinegar, olive oil, borax, and lemon juice (be sure to dispose of toxic items safely). For safer cleaning in the home, use these "recipes for healthy household cleaners," adapted from *Creative Reuse Extravaganza*, by Cynthia Ashley and Sylvia Valazques.

- **All Purpose Cleaner:** Place undiluted white vinegar into a spray bottle. You will be amazed at what it will clean, and it will not harm surfaces.
- **Carpet Freshener:** Sprinkle baking soda over the carpet. Let it sit for several hours, then vacuum it. Like baking soda placed in the refrigerator, it will absorb unwanted odors.
- **Floor and Furniture Polish:** Mix one part lemon juice and two parts olive oil, and pour into a container; shake. Pour a small amount onto furniture or the floor and rub well using a rag. (Reconstituted lemon juice will do just fine; if you are going to use fresh lemons, strain the pulp and seeds out before mixing with the olive oil.)
- **Laundry Bleach:** Add one-half cup of white vinegar, baking soda, or borax to each load. It will act as a bleach for dingy, dirty clothes without harming them.
- **Moth Repellent:** Place a handful of cedar chips and/or lavender flowers in a small square of netting, or a sheer material such as old nylons or pantyhose, to make a sachet. Tie it closed with wire or ribbon and hang in your closet or place in drawers to keep moths away.
- **Toilet Bowl Cleaner:** Sprinkle baking soda or borax into the toilet bowl. Add a small amount of white vinegar. Scrub with a toilet brush.
- **Window Cleaner:** Mix one part white vinegar with one part water and pour into a spray bottle. If the

smell of vinegar is too strong, mix one part vinegar and two parts water. Even diluted, the mixture is still an effective window cleaner.

Water Filtration Systems

If you are concerned about safe drinking water, there is hope in point-of-use filtration systems that employ a water filter at the kitchen faucet. (See Chapter 6 for more on dirty drinking water.) Your greatest exposure to chlorine, however, is not from drinking water but from taking showers. If you like taking baths and you want to protect yourself from the chlorine in the bath water, you can do what friends of mine do. They heat up filtered water on the stove and transport the heated water into their tub in big pots. If you don't want to work that hard, consider whole-house filtration or a point-of-use filter in the bathroom. Fortunately, there are several high-quality water purification systems on the market. When looking at buying a water filtration unit for your home, consider these six factors:

1. Does it take out all or most of the toxic compounds that could be harmful to your health?
2. Does it leave in beneficial minerals?
3. Is it cost-effective?
4. Is it easy to install and maintain?
5. Is it friendly to the environment?
6. Does the filtered water taste good?

According to Dr. Jeffrey Bland, a nutritional biochemist, the best water purification systems include pre- and post-compressed charcoal filters with a reverse osmosis

(RO) membrane in between the two charcoal filters. During the water filtration process, water first goes into a pre-charcoal filter, then through the RO membrane, and finally through the post-charcoal filter. These filtration units must be placed below the sink and usually are installed by a plumber. Because they contain more working parts than other types of water filters, they are more costly to purchase and maintain, but they are often available at discount buying clubs. They also use up approximately one gallon of water for every gallon that they purify. The charcoal filters must be replaced every six months, adding to the solid waste in our landfills.

Doulton, producer of some of the world's best china, makes a simpler unit that is available in above- or below-counter models. Doulton's basic unit is a three-stage filter molded into a single cartridge. The first stage is a diatomaceous earth ceramic that traps 99.99 percent of bacteria and cysts, according to their literature. The second and third stages, which combine a zeolite metal ion reduction medium, granular carbon, and powdered carbon in a tightly packed matrix, filter out toxic chemicals (chlorine, pesticides, solvents, etc.) and heavy metals (lead, aluminum, etc.); such beneficial minerals as calcium and magnesium are left in the water.

The Doulton filter is one of the most effective and economical water filters I have found. The maintenance on this unit is easy: you simply remove the plastic housing and use your vegetable brush to scrub off the collected debris. The minimum advertised life of the cartridge is one year, based on a family of four using the system daily, though some would dispute the effectiveness of the carbon portion of the filter beyond six months. (For ordering information, see Appendix 1.)

A word of warning about the hand-held pitcher-type water filters advertised nationally, which consist of only granular carbon particles: These filters may actually increase your exposure to disease-producing microorganisms. In time, the tap water no longer comes in contact with the charcoal granules because channels are formed as the water repeatedly runs through the unit. Eventually, residue from previously filtered water collects on these channels and acts as a breeding ground for harmful microorganisms.

You may need to add additional stages to an under the counter filter depending on the harmful solvents in your water supply. Whatever type of filter you buy, make sure that you can get an ongoing supply of replacement filters, since the effectiveness of water filters is dependent on regular maintenance. (For more information, see Appendix 1.)

HOUSEHOLD PESTICIDES

Did you ever consider that mowing your lawn could be hazardous to your health? An article in the October 14, 1991, *Wall Street Journal* reported the case of Tom Latimer, a vigorous, athletic man with a bright future as a petroleum engineer. After one hour of cutting the grass, picking up clippings, and edging the walkways around his home one Saturday morning, he felt dizzy and nauseated. His nose was running and his chest was tight. He had a pounding headache. Ten days later, he was still getting sicker. He suffered with constant head pain, and his eyes began to jerk uncontrollably. Within months, he developed testicular cancer. Six years and twenty doctors later, Latimer accepted the diagnosis that he was poisoned by an organophosphate pesticide used to treat his yard. Earlier that summer he had sprayed a different organophosphate on some ant hills and insect nests in his yard.

Normally, the liver can detoxify small amounts of a pesticide in one or two days, but Latimer had a complicating factor: he was taking Tagamet, which is generally prescribed to control excessive stomach acid. Alfredo Sadun, Ph.D., a professor of neurosurgery and ophthalmology at the University of Southern California, says that taking a medication such as Tagamet "can make a person 100 to 1,000 times more sensitive to organophosphate poisoning." Tagamet and NSAIDs (non-steroidal anti-inflammatory drugs), such as Aleve, Motrin, Tylenol, and aspirin, interfere with the cytochrome P450 pathway—the liver's first phase of detoxification.

Latimer and his wife had both worked in the yard in bare arms and shorts, digging around flower beds and shrubbery that were treated with the pesticide. His wife wasn't taking Tagamet, and she didn't get sick.

Tom Latimer can no longer ride a bike. He has difficulty walking. At night, to combat brain seizures and nightmares, he takes an anti-epileptic medicine. His sleep is disturbed. And annual laser surgery has to be performed to remove viral growths on his vocal cords due to immunosuppression caused by xenobiotic exposure. His home and work life have been damaged. With Latimer's natural defenses compromised by the combination of NSAIDs, Tagamet, and pesticides, the poison carried out a potent and ongoing attack on his nervous system.

A growing body of research indicates that many Americans may be vulnerable to chronic, low-level exposure to pesticides, which can produce severe abdominal pain, headaches, nausea, and other effects. Recent estimates suggest that each year there are 3,000,000 severe pesticide poisonings (including accidents such as spills, unprotected agriculture application, factory, explosions, etc.) and 220,000 deaths worldwide. In the United States, pesticide-related illnesses are estimated to occur between 150,000 and 300,000 times a year. Over time, the risks from exposure vary depending on a number of factors such as individual sensitivity levels and immune suppression, but may include cancer, birth defects, and damage to the liver, kidneys, and nervous system.

In an October 1994 article in *Medical Hypothesis* titled "Neurasthenic Fatigue, Chemical Sensitivity, and GABA Receptor Toxins," F. M. Corrigan and S. MacDonald reported that low levels of insecticides and polychlorinated biphenyls (PCBs) found in our environment and the body fat of humans may be the cause of chronic fatigue syndromes, including multiple chemical sensitivities in susceptible individuals. Other symptoms and disorders caused by exposure to pesticides and PCBs include: throat irritation and dryness, bouts of profuse sweating, headaches, muscle pains, weakness, concentration difficulties, joint pains, palpitations, chest pain and tightness, reduced tolerance for alcohol, dizziness, elevated Epstein-Barr titer, cognitive dysfunction, back pain, swollen glands, hypersensitivity to light, decreased appetite, sleepiness, anxiety, atrial fibrillation, irritability, indecisiveness, depression, personality change, and flu-like symptoms. Elevated Epstein-Barr titer is closely associated with Chronic Fatigue Immunodeficiency Syndrome (CFIDS).

The problem with public warnings about such risks is that neither the Food and Drug Administration (FDA) nor the Environmental Protection Agency (EPA) test for toxicity from combined chemicals, even those commonly used together. Testing for the effects of combinations of medications and chemicals is far beyond their reach.

In the June 1996, issue of *Science* magazine, a group of researchers from Tulane University reported in their article "Synergistic Activation of Estrogen Receptor with Combinations of Environmental Chemicals" on a preliminary investigation into the effect of combined pesticides that by themselves have little effect on the activity of estrogen. When combined, however, their stimulation of estrogen receptors and activity was increased. A surplus of estrogen has been linked to breast cancer and malformation of male sex organs. John A. McLachlan, principal investigator, said, "If you test them individually, you could conclude that they were nonestrogenic, almost inconsequential. But when we put them in combination, their potency jumped up 500- to 1000-fold."

In *Our Stolen Future*, authors Theo Colborn, Dianne Dumanovski, and John Peterson Myers state, "Hormonally active synthetic chemicals are thugs on the biological information highway that sabotage vital communication. They mug the messengers or impersonate them. They jam signals. They scramble messages. They sow disinformation. They wreak all manner of havoc." And this havoc seems to spread across generations.

Since PCBs show up in our water supplies and the fish that swim in them, Helen Daly and a team of researchers at State University of New York at Oswego fed rats a diet that included salmon from nearby Lake Ontario in 1992. They found behavioral problems; when confronted with mildly negative situations, the fish-fed rats became "hyper-reactive," in Daly's words. Not only were the rat pups affected, but the mother's behavior was also abnormal. Even more startling was the finding that the mother rat's grandchildren overreacted as well. This is very significant. Even though the second and third generation rats were not exposed to PCBs, they suffered damage as a consequence of the first generation female's exposure. (The same results have been seen with nutritional deficiency. The offspring for two generations show signs of zinc deficiency including a weakened immune system. Even receiving sufficient quantities of zinc cannot make up for their grandmother's zinc deficiency. Adult humans need from 40 to 80 milligrams of zinc in their diet per day.) Daly has shown that this cross-generational effect is not gender biased, at least in rats. And in May of 1995, the Oswego team announced that they had found similar behavioral effects in human children.

As we have seen, pesticides and other *xenobiotics* (chemical compounds that are foreign to a living organism) can affect the sex hormones in your body. Depending on the chemical, they may stimulate hormone production, or they may lower hormone levels by accelerating their breakdown and elimination, thereby leaving your body short not only of estrogen, but of testosterone and other hormones as well. Hormones are produced by endocrine glands, including the thyroid, thymus, pancreas, adrenals, ovaries, and testicles. Hormones regulate a multitude of functions, including brain development, energy level, immune-system function, sugar metabolism, stress response, bone strength, sex drive, sexual characteristics, and fertility. The adrenal glands, which produce stress hormones, are affected by xenobiotic compounds more than any other organ, followed by the thyroid gland.

Many of us know about the temperature-regulating effects of the thyroid gland and how the activity of the thyroid determines our basal and resting metabolic rates, which in turn influence your weight. But the thyroid is also needed in the development of the brain. Research has shown that thyroid hormones stimulate the production and placement of nerve cells within the brain. Pesticides such as PCBs and dioxins mimic or block this hormone action. Problems resulting from interference with your natural hormones range from mental retardation to behavioral disorders such as hyperactivity and learning disabilities such as Attention Deficit Disorder (ADD).

A severe example of pesticide poisoning is seen in the children born to Taiwanese women who ate cooking oil that was accidentally contaminated with high levels of PCBs and furans. Furans are flammable liquids made synthetically or from the wood oils of pine. They have toxic effects similar to dioxins, of which the most infamous is Agent Orange used in the Vietnam War. Dioxin has earned its reputation as *the* most dangerous synthetic chemical as a result of the damage soldiers exposed to Agent Orange suffered, ranging from cancer to handicaps in their offspring. (We are now seeing the negative health effects of agents used in Desert Storm. According to Dr. Jeffrey Bland there were ". . . an unexpected number of suicides in the returning vets who were still ill." Dr. Bland has submitted a grant to the government to help these unfortunate soldiers with effective therapies to detoxify the poisons to which they were exposed.)

The children of the Taiwanese women exposed to PCBs and furans suffered a range of health defects, including the sexual organ effects we have become familiar with from investigation of other hormone-stimulating xenobiotics. For instance, boys exposed to PCBs and furans have a significantly shorter penis than boys of the same age not exposed. In general, the children showed permanent impairment in their motor and coordination skills and mental abilities. Behavioral problems including hyperactivity made it difficult for them to concentrate and to learn.

Children whose mothers ate Lake Michigan fish during their pregnancies showed similar effects. The women ate the fish only twice per month in the six years prior to pregnancy, and some had none while pregnant. The more fish the mother ate, the smaller was her baby's head, which suggests decreased brain size and intelligence. The babies also had a lower birth weight than did the group who had consumed no fish. They exhibited weak reflexes and more jerky movements. At seven months, they showed impaired cognitive function, which includes all aspects of perceiving, thinking, and remembering. And at four years of age, the children of women with the highest PCB levels had lower scores in verbal and memory tests. In both groups of children—the Taiwanese and the Lake Michigan—the chemicals their mothers were exposed to interfered with the thyroid's ability to optimally organize their brains while they were developing in the womb.

Alternatives to Toxic Pesticides

Use natural pest control. Ask your local organic farmers, contact your local library, or check with your local nursery for alternatives to dangerous chemical pesticides. I use McKenzie Rock Flour to keep my plants healthy (see Appendix 1 for more information). Like humans, if plants are fed the proper nutrients they will have greater resistance to disease.

To rid your home of such pests as ants and cockroaches, diatomaceous earth works well. Diatomaceous earth is a natural pesticide that works by mechanical action instead of chemical action. This avoids the problem of pests that adapt by mutating into resistant future generations, as is the case with chemical pesticides. Diatomaceous earth can be used to de-worm your animals—especially horses.

To deal with termite infestation, there is a type of worm, called a nematode, that parasitizes and kills termites. (Note that the nematode treatment cannot be applied in areas where termite sprays have been previously used.) Other less toxic methods for dealing with termites include electricity, heat treatment, and freezing. You can also find safe alternatives to pesticides in the Gardens Alive! catalog and from the Bio-Integral Resource Center (BIRC) organization in Berkeley (see Appendix 1).

MERCURY AMALGAM FILLINGS

Modern dentistry can correct the effects of bad diet and improper oral hygiene by drilling and filling cavities, performing root canals, and providing caps and bridges. But there appear to be risks from dental procedures. Many cutting-edge dentists are seeing the ill effects of "silver" ("silver" fillings contain mercury and other metal and nonmetal compounds) or mercury amalgam fillings and metal posts that are secured into the jaw in root canals.

Mercury amalgam fillings may be a significant factor contributing to bad health. Dr. Jeffrey Bland recommends that anyone with adult acne, neurological problems, or autoimmune disorders consider working with a dentist who specializes in removing mercury amalgam fillings and replacing them with composite fillings. Other symptoms of mercury toxicity, according to Dr. Michael Lebowitz, a chiropractor who specializes in helping the chronically ill, are depression, memory loss, food sensitivities, and "weird neuropathies." *Neuropathies*—functional disturbances or pathological changes in the peripheral nervous system— usually manifest as unusual sensations in the arms and legs, such as numbness and tingling.

In Europe, the problem of amalgam use is being taken seriously in professional circles. Countries such as Sweden and Austria have restricted or eliminated the use of amalgam fillings, and Germany's leading supplier of amalgam is getting out of the market. For the sake of patients, dentists, and dental assistants, mercury amalgam will be replaced by other materials before too long.

In the United States in 1994, approximately six percent of dentists recognized the danger of mercury amalgam fillings. Since this is a recently recognized danger, your dentist may not know much about the topic. The American Dental Association's stance is that there are no dangers associated with this material, and they make no moves to restrict its use.

Unfortunately, the time of greatest exposure to mercury besides filling is during removal. If you are going to have your fillings removed and replaced with composite material, I recommend that you contact a professional consultant (see Appendix 1). Some people have complete immune system breakdowns after having their fillings taken out. Here are a few precautions you should take to minimize your risk:

1. Make sure your whole mouth is covered with a rubber dam during removal.
2. Wear a mask or get oxygen during the procedure.
3. Have a shot of DMPS, a complexing agent, within twelve to twenty-four hours before removal.

(DMPS takes the mercury out of your body through urine.)

Sources of toxins present themselves in many ways and from many fronts. To effectively reduce your toxic load, you must first be able to recognize where they came from in order for you to minimize their impact on your life. Since you cannot completely escape toxic exposure, cleansing programs are essential to improve your health. See Parts 3 and 4 for help finding your way safely through our polluted world.

CHAPTER 6

Environmental Toxins

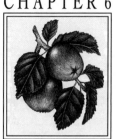

It is virtually impossible to escape toxic substances. Air goes everywhere. Water evaporates into the atmosphere, circulates, and rains down onto the earth's surface, where it drains into streams, rivers, and oceans. Strong air and water currents carry pollution to the farthest reaches of the north and south poles.

How Environmental Toxins Move Up the Food Chain

Humans eat at the top of the food chain, which means eating other animals, birds, and fish, as opposed to eating plants and algae exclusively. Like humans, plants and animals store toxins in their fatty parts. Toxins move up the food chain from plants, bugs, and algae, to a small fish or mammal, which is then eaten by a large fish or mammal, which is consumed by a human. Toxins are also passed on to a newborn

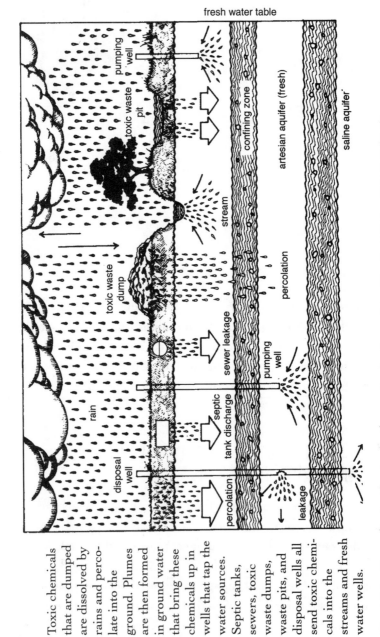

Toxic chemicals that are dumped are dissolved by rains and percolate into the ground. Plumes are then formed in ground water that bring these chemicals up in wells that tap the water sources. Septic tanks, sewers, toxic waste dumps, waste pits, and disposal wells all send toxic chemicals into the streams and fresh water wells.

Figure 6.1 Groundwater Contamination   (Reprinted by permission of Jon Goodchild from *Well Body, Well Earth.*)

through mother's milk. At each level of the food chain, the toxins become more concentrated (see Figure 6.1).

The May 13, 1996, *Los Angeles Times* carried an article about the effect of pollution on the human immune system. The Inuit people of Arctic Canada, although far from industrialization, are believed to be the most highly contaminated humans on earth. The world's pollution is carried to them on northbound air and ocean currents and in the native foods that they eat. These Native Americans eat mostly fish and marine mammals, whose bodies carry a high concentration of fat, to protect them from frigid arctic waters and from starvation when food is scarce. Because of this, they are exposed to the maximum concentration of toxins in their diet.

Perhaps the most tragic part of the story is that the toxins accumulated in the bodies of the fish and marine mammals concentrate even more in a mother's milk. The *Los Angeles Times* reported that Inuit babies have low B- and T-cell counts from immune system suppression caused by feeding on their mother's breast milk, which has a high concentration of PCBs and DDT. (B- and T-cells are produced by the body's cells and thymus gland, respectively, in response to invading microorganisms.) PCBs are used to insulate electrical transformers far from Broughton Island where the Inuit live, and DDT is used thousands of miles away from their Canadian Arctic region. Yet these dangerous chemicals reach the Eskimos and are then passed onto their children. Inuit children take in seven times more PCBs than the typical infant in southern Canada or the United States. A 1995 study found abnormalities in the immune systems of these children, including the discovery that their bodies do not produce the necessary antibodies when they

are vaccinated for smallpox, measles, polio, and other diseases. The increased rate of infection also leads to loss of
hearing in one out of four children.

POLLUTION AND IMMUNOSUPPRESSION

Pollution, however, is not restricted to the north pole. Children who live near tanning factories in the southern part of
the United States have a higher rate of leukemia than the general population. Many of the survivors of the radiation explo-
sion at Chernobyl in the former USSR need bone marrow
transplants to produce red blood cells just to stay alive. In the
Los Angeles Times article referred to above, Steve Hollanday,
an immunotoxicologist at Virginia-Maryland Regional College of Veterinary Medicine, states, "We're probably all—and
I mean the whole doggone planet—immunosuppressed." *Immunosuppression* is a condition in which the body does not have
the strength and resilience to fight off bacteria, viruses, and
parasites. As a result, cells that have been damaged by pollution and drugs will not be recognized and destroyed. If damaged cells are not destroyed they may multiply and divide,
reproducing themselves as mutated cells which may in turn
develop into cancer.

FALLING SPERM COUNTS

Men should pay particular attention to the following information about chemical effects that decrease male potency
and cause malformation of male sex organs. Sperm counts
are dropping for all species across the planet. To count
sperm, we measure millions of sperm per milliliter of semen.
In the past five decades, the count has been dropping by

approximately one million sperm per milliliter each year. Since 1938, with the rise of industrialization, human male sperm count has dropped by half. To have the pool from which future generations will emerge cut in half in only fifty years is a shocking threat to the future of humanity. Studies from Scotland, Belgium, and France in the early 90s showed an inverse correlation between the year of birth and the health of a man's sperm. Men born in 1945 and measured in 1975 averaged 102 million sperm per milliliter of semen. Men born in 1962 and measured in 1992 averaged 51 million. If this trend continues, by the year 2005 a thirty-year-old man would have a sperm count equaling just twenty-five percent of that of the average male born in 1925. If we don't change our lifestyle, will men be producing any sperm by the year 2042?

The quantity of sperm is not the only factor we need to consider. As we move forward in time, more sperm are deformed and miss their target because they don't swim right; the incidence of testicular cancer has jumped sharply, and genital abnormalities such as undescended testicles and shortened urinary tracts are on the rise. This is a problem *and* there is a way out of the dilemma through cleansing and lifestyle changes.

One way to decrease exposure to pollutants and their negative effects on your health and sperm count is to eat organic fruit and vegetables. A recent Danish study, which compared farmers to airline workers, was reported in the June 30, 1996, issue of the *San Francisco Examiner.* Each group was analyzed for their sperm count. The group of organic farmers, at least one-quarter of whose diet is pesticide-free produce, were found to have sperm counts forty-three percent higher than the airline workers.

Pesticides are designed to kill living things. And much to the distress of our health and fertility as a species, our bodies mistake these xenobiotic compounds for our own estrogens. Estrogen is a hormone that is responsible for creating female characteristics. Males exposed to increasing amounts of estrogenic compounds are being feminized by a lowered ratio of testosterone to estrogen, and possibly because receptor sites for male hormones are blocked by estrogenic substances. Testosterone is a hormone in greater concentration in men that is responsible for male sexual and behavioral characteristics. *The San Francisco Examiner* article goes on further to state other factors which may be involved in decreasing sperm counts. These factors correspond to greater exposure to other harmful chemicals through city living vs. country living and eating processed vs. whole foods.

DIRTY WATER

Often you hear news reports about a new contamination problem in the water supplies throughout the United States. According to the U.S. Environmental Protection Agency (EPA), there are nearly 200,000 active surface impoundments (ground level collection sites) in the United States, of which about 26,000 are unlined and may be leaking a wide variety of toxic chemicals into underground water supplies. John Skinner, a director of the EPA's Office of Solid Waste Programs, reported in a congressional hearing that ninety-five percent of all operating surface impoundments are located within a quarter mile of drinking water supplies. Once ground water has become contaminated, it is almost impossible to purify.

Beginning on December 1, 1996, the *San Francisco Examiner* did a three-part series on water quality, and reported: "The nation's drinking water is at risk." Water pipes are aging, population is booming, and germs in our water are becoming more resistant to the chemicals traditionally used to kill them. In 1993, 403,000 people in Milwaukee got sick and 104 died from contamination by the microbe cryptosporidium. The same year, residents of New York City and Washington, D.C., were warned to boil their water before drinking it because it contained E. coli (fecal bacteria). Since then, at least 850 other community water systems have been ordered to boil their water. In 1995, the U.S. Centers for Disease Control and Prevention (CDC) advised people with weakened immune systems, such as those with AIDS or who have undergone chemotherapy or organ transplants, to boil water, to use filters or drink certain bottled waters. (Contact the CDC in Atlanta, Georgia, for more information, 404-639-3311.)

In February of 1996, a judge in Austin, Texas, levied $915,000 in penalties against a water company. One witness against the company testified that the water from his faucet caught fire when he placed a candle near it.

The EPA makes water safety rules and the states are responsible for enforcing them. However, they rarely take action against utilities in violation. When the states do not intervene, the EPA is supposed to step in. Both say they have insufficient funds to get tough against offenders. The General Accounting Office, the investigative branch of Congress, repeatedly finds problems. A 1990 investigation revealed that states take action against only one-fourth of the utilities that chronically violate EPA standards. They found that, of those water companies that violate standards, almost half of them do so for more than four years before any action is taken. Some of these violations pose serious health risks. In 1995 alone, close to 9,000 violations of contaminant levels in community drinking water were exposed.

It is important to drink *pure* water. Why do I stress pure water as opposed to just water? At a recent meeting of Health in Common, an organization of consumers and health care providers, I had the opportunity to hear a presentation by Larry Colb from the California State Water Quality Control Board. When questioned as to the number of chemical substances for which California's state-of-the-art water treatment facilities test, we were told, "about seventy or so." Yet each year, as we learned from our Surgeon General as early as 1979, one thousand new man-made chemicals are released into the environment. Our modern water purification systems are testing for less than ten percent of the possible pollutants that are produced annually. The seventy or so that are tested for also exclude the thousand or more chemicals that were introduced last year and the thousand or more produced and released the year before and the year before that.

The problem with water is even more insidious than synthetic chemicals in our environment winding up in our water supply, because the chlorine that is used to disinfect drinking water is in itself harmful and dangerous when mixed with organic residues in the water we consume. Several primate studies link drinking water to bowel and bladder cancer. Trihalomethanes formed by the chemical bonding of chlorine with organic residues in water are known carcinogens. Some water treatment facilities are aware of this problem and work to reduce levels by adding ammonia to the water after the chlorine has sat for a while. When ammonia is added, the chlorine preferentially bonds to the ammonia, thus reducing the formation of carcinogens. For most people, these levels will not create an immediate health risk, but we simply don't know what the effect may be over time. For populations of the young, old, and/or sick, these small effects may add up to dysfunction and disease.

Toxic Plumbing

Next, we must consider the pipes that deliver water to our faucets and the material from which the faucets are made. There is concern about lead entering the water from solder and faucets. According to a February 1997 report from the EPA, ninety-one percent of the lead that contaminates domestic water is leached from the plumbing, rather than coming from the water source. Many are familiar with the toxic effects that exposure to lead in house paints can have on childhood brain development such as learning disabilities requiring remedial education, impaired visual-motor development, damage to the nervous and immune systems and behavioral problems.

Some homes have copper water-supply pipes. Copper ions from the pipes can leach into the water supply. A 1995 report, "The Need to Revise the National Drinking Water Regulations for Copper" (*Regul Toxicology Pharmacology*), by K. S. Sidhu Prom recommends that the level of copper in our drinking water should be reduced. Infants and children up to ten years old have an increased susceptibility to copper toxicity due to the normal elevation of copper level in their livers and the lack of mechanisms to regulate it in their bodies. Adverse effects of copper toxicity are abdominal pain, nausea, vomiting, diarrhea, headaches, and dizziness.

Faced with the facts of poor water quality, the point-of-use water filtration system for your kitchen faucet makes sense. (For more information on water filters, see Chapter 5 and refer to Appendix 1.)

TOXIC OVERLOAD

In September of 1991, the EPA published a report entitled *Toxics in the Community: The 1989 Toxics Release Inventory (TRI) National Report*, which yielded some staggering figures. The largest toxic releases involved twenty-five chemicals, and totaled 5,705,670,380 pounds. Of this 5.7 billion pounds, 42.5 percent went into the air, 3.3 percent were released into surface water, 7.8 percent were on land, 20.7 percent flowed into underground water, 9.6 percent joined with public sewage, and 16 percent were off-site (brought to other places such as surface impoundments). Among the twenty-five toxic substances were: toluene, a known carcinogen commonly found in nail polish; sulfuric acid, a poison to lungs and mucous membranes; and freon, which destroys the ozone layer and causes increased exposure to excess ultraviolet rays, increasing the risk of skin cancer.

Although PCBs have been banned in the United States since 1976, nothing was done to limit the use of PCBs already manufactured, so we continue to suffer the consequences of exposure. And *dioxins* continue to be released into our environment as a result of the production of pesticides and wood preservatives, bleaching paper to become white, burning trash that contains plastics and paper, and burning fossil fuels (cooking and driving automobiles).

How to Avoid Dioxins

But don't despair. There are immediate, effective steps you can take to minimize or eliminate most risks of living in an industrialized world. Here are some alternatives to the dioxin-producing processes (also see Appendix 1):

- Avoid the use of pesticides on your lawn, and talk to neighbors about doing the same.
- Talk to your local hardware store about carrying dioxin-free wood preservatives.
- Buy unbleached paper products for your kitchen and bathroom.
- If your trash is burned, separate out plastics and paper for recycling.
- Eat more raw fruits and vegetables if your digestion permits (if not, cook them as lightly as possible and/or consult a specialist to help you improve your digestion).
- Drive less, walk more, ride a bicycle, or carpool.

Hormone Disruption

In July of 1991 a prestigious group of scientists—including experts in anthropology, ecology, toxicology, law, psychiatry, wildlife management, medicine, and related fields—met because they were concerned about the hormone-disrupting effects of substances like diethylstilbestrol (DES) in the environment. Their meeting produced what is called "The Wingspread Consensus Statement." On the subject of "Chemically-Induced Alterations in Sexual Development: The Wildlife/Human Connection," they stated with certainty: "The effects seen in *in utero* DES-exposed humans parallel those found in contaminated wildlife and laboratory animals, suggesting that humans may be at risk to the same environmental hazards as wildlife."

Endocrine specialists have found little difference among the hormone functions of most species that inhabit the earth. What happens to one species hormonally happens to all species. I interpret their statement to mean that we cannot ignore the disappearance of our Great Lakes mink populations, or the problems observed in bird populations: eggs that don't hatch; deformities such as crossed bills, missing eyes, and clubbed feet; and abnormal nesting behavior. Nor can we ignore the fact that our St. Lawrence River beluga whale population is now a mere five hundred, down from five thousand at the turn of the century, that eighty percent of the sanderling bird population dropped in a fifteen-year period, or that half the population of bottlenose dolphins that migrate along the eastern seaboard were lost to sickness from pesticide-induced immune system suppression.

Some explain the disappearance of wildlife from the planet with reasons other than xenobiotic poisoning, such as habitat destruction, overkill, and species competition. However, these cannot account for the pathologies found during autopsy of dead fish, birds, and mammals. Beluga whales on autopsy had malignant tumors, benign tumors, breast tumors, abdominal masses, bladder cancer, emphysema, and ulcers of the mouth, esophagus, stomach, and intestines. Most had severe gum disease and missing teeth. Many had pneumonia or viral and bacterial infections. More than half the females had breast infections, making it impossible to feed their young. Others had endocrine disorders, including enlargement of the thyroid gland and cysts in the thyroid. Some had twisted spines and other skeletal disorders. Xenobiotic poisoning has been shown to be the cause of many of these disorders. We live on this planet with those diseased and deformed fish, birds, and mammals. It is unlikely that we humans can escape exposure to the same environmental poisons that damage our wildlife, since we share the same earth, air, and water. We do, however, have a more sure way of recovery with detoxification.

PART III:
INTERNAL
CLEANSING

CHAPTER 7

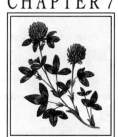

DIETARY FIBER FOR GOOD HEALTH

My grandmother used to tell me to eat my roughage (also called crude fiber—the cellulose or cell wall of plants). Scientists have found other equally active components of fiber, including cellulose, hemicellulose, pectin, lignan, gums, and mucilages. Dietary fiber has been defined as the substances in food that are not digested and absorbed in the small intestines.

The FDA has set a Recommended Daily Allowance (RDA) for dietary fiber of 25 grams per day for a 2,000-calorie diet. If you take in less or more than 2,000 calories a day, as many Americans do, they recommend adjusting the amount of fiber accordingly. The standard Western diet contains only 10 to 20 grams of fiber per day, while research points to the necessity of at least 40 to 60 grams per day for good health. The FDA came only halfway with its recommendation for optimal fiber intake, but it is a definite improvement over no recommendation at all. Low fiber intake is one of the reasons there is such an urgent need for internal cleansing in Western countries.

Fiber comes in many forms. For most people, the best way to get adequate fiber is to eat lots of fruit and vegetables. Sadly, most Americans get most of their fiber from white bread. Knowing this, it is not surprising to learn that Americans are sorely deficient in this important dietary component. In their book *The Omega-3 Phenomenon*, nutritionist Clara Felix and Donald Rudin, M.D., note that the fiber content of white bread is less than one gram per slice. The American Dietetic Association recommends five servings of fruits and vegetables per day. One serving equals one cup of raw, or one-half cup of cooked, fruit or vegetables.

In summarizing their review of the scientific literature on dietary fiber, Martin A. Eastwood and R. Passmore, fiber researchers who followed up on Dr. Denis Burkitt's work, concluded in the *Lancet:* "It can be stated with confidence that people who increase their fiber intake up to 50 grams per day [which is] double the amount usually present in British [and other Western] diets run no risk of any serious adverse effects on their health." Some reports have stated that very high-fiber diets, especially those with high wheat bran content, may tend to bind some minerals and thus reduce their absorption in the body.

FIBER SUPPLEMENTS

If you are concerned about mineral absorption, choose fiber supplements other than wheat bran. I use three fiber supplements in my office: Colon Care Formula (CCF) by Yerba Prima, Ultra Fiber (UF) by HealthComm, and Nutri Flax (NF) by Omega Nutrition. Colon Care Formula and Ultra

Fiber are combinations of soluble and insoluble fibers for optimal effect. Ultra Fiber has no psyllium husks in it for persons who have a sensitivity to this form of fiber. It does, however, have a high concentration of barley fiber, which can be problematic for some sensitive individuals. Nutri Flax is powdered flaxseed that has been specially prepared to ensure freshness and effectiveness. If there is a concern regarding cancer risk, this would be my fiber of choice since flax fiber promotes the production of mammalian lignan, which has a potent anticancer effect. It is very helpful to have three high-quality therapeutic options for people who need a fiber supplement.

Fiber Improves Bowel Function

With an increase in daily fiber intake, you will typically be immediately aware of an improvement in bowel function. Dietary fiber—in particular the hemicellulose portion—absorbs water in the intestines to provide bulk and soften the stools. This makes for less straining with bowel movements. The hemicellulose type of fiber is essential because of its ability to absorb released toxins and aid in elimination from the body.

Fiber Decreases Transit Time

Increased daily fiber intake will decrease the time it takes for the food you eat to pass through your twenty to thirty feet of intestinal tubing and be eliminated in a bowel movement. It takes approximately ten hours for food to pass into the colon, but the amount of time it sits in the colon can vary dramatically. While the normal range of total transit time for people on a high-fiber diet is ten to fifty hours, people on a Western diet have an average transit time of sixty-five to one hundred hours. For most of those hours, the partially digested food (now your body's waste material) sits in the colon being worked on by disease-producing yeasts and bacteria. Normal transit time is a health blessing because environmental and dietary toxins have less time to come in contact with the colon lining and therefore less chance to be reabsorbed into your blood stream (see "Food Transit Times" on page 24).

Fiber Normalizes the Bowel

Paradoxically, fiber is also helpful for people who have an irritable bowel with loose, frequent, and perhaps urgent bowel movements. It helps both with constipation or sluggish bowel movements and diarrhea or loose bowel movements.

Fiber Lowers Cholesterol Levels

Studies have shown that some fibers, such as psyllium husks, pectin, oat and rice bran, and guar gum, have a cholesterol-lowering effect on the blood. They lower the level of harmful LDL cholesterol in the body, while raising the valuable and protective HDL cholesterol level. One man I know found that after daily use of psyllium husks for four months (two teaspoons per day), his cholesterol count dropped from 260 to under 200, the lowest it had ever been. This change in his cholesterol from the simple addition of dietary fiber took his heart attack risk back down into the normal range.

Fiber Protects Against Chronic Degenerative Disease

Over the years, daily fiber intake will protect against the risk of a number of chronic diseases. Its antitoxic properties, its ability to nourish the growth of beneficial intestinal bacteria such as lactobacillus, its sweeping action in the colon, and its swelling action, which results in softer and bulkier stools, all contribute to long-term health. Research findings worldwide led the director of the Division of Cancer Prevention and Control at the National Cancer Institute to issue a statement in August of 1984 recommending that Americans eat a diet high in fiber to reduce the risk of colon and rectal cancer (the third highest cause of cancer deaths in the United States, according to the American Cancer Society in 1992). The many benefits of dietary fiber are summarized in Figure 3.2 on page 39.

Fiber Normalizes Blood Sugar

Fiber slows the release of sugar into your bloodstream, which prevents an exhausting demand for the release of insulin. If you have normal pancreatic function, your body produces insulin in response to the sugar load in your bloodstream from food you have eaten. Insulin brings your blood levels back into a normal range. Diabetics who cannot produce insulin from their pancreas must use medication in tablet form or by injection to normalize their blood sugar. As a benefit of adequate fiber intake, insulin-dependent diabetics may be able to reduce their required dose of insulin. If you do have diabetes, decrease your insulin intake only under the supervision of your medical doctor to assure your safety. Hypoglycemic individuals can maintain a more stable blood sugar level and prevent peaks and valleys in their daily energy by including more fiber in their diet.

A HISTORY OF BREAKFAST FIBER IN AMERICA

The history of modern interest in good nutrition as it relates to health is intertwined with fiber cereals and eating a good breakfast. This is hard to imagine when you step into the cereal aisle of your local supermarket. Row after row of bright, colorful, sugar-laden cereals nearly jump off the shelves and into your cart. When children are along on a shopping trip, the sugar cereals they have seen advertised on their cartoon shows usually succeed in making it into the cart. Of course, adults are not immune to this siren call. Yet more adults are picking up high-fiber cereals such as Kellogg's All Bran, Post Raisin Bran, and Quaker Oat Bran. This brings us back to our nineteenth-century roots.

Breakfast was not always considered a distinct meal. The first concepts of breakfast date back to the 1400s. Then it was usually a high-fat, high-calorie meal geared toward heavy agricultural or manual labor. Agricultural workers may have been able to use up all of those calories throughout the day, but can you?

The transition took place over time in the 1800s and early 1900s. Graham crackers are named after health pioneer Sylvester Graham, who in the mid-1800s stressed the importance of whole-meal bread with the fiber intact. Seventh Day Adventists followed up on Graham's teachings. One very influential advocate, Sister Ellen White, began the

Battle Creek Sanitarium in Battle Creek, Michigan, in the late 1800s. She taught the value of whole grains and vegetarian diet for good health. One of the early whole grain cereals served at the sanitarium was called Granose Flakes.

Two of the employees at the Battle Creak Sanitarium were W.K. Kellogg and John Harvey Kellogg. In the world of cereals, there is no name more famous than Kellogg. The Kellogg company began in 1906 with Kellogg's Corn Flakes. To this day, Kellogg's Corn Flakes remains the top-selling cereal in the world. Their best-known high-fiber cereal, All Bran, began in 1916 as Krumbled Bran and was changed to its current name in 1923. You and I both know why people eat All Bran. Until 1941, the label was quite explicit: It said right on the box, "Relieves Constipation."

Kellogg's All Bran is known for one more breakthrough, though, in the 1980s. With the cooperation of the National Cancer Institute, Kellogg's began an educational campaign on the back of All Bran boxes describing the link between high-fiber diets and reduced risk of cancer. Sales of All Bran doubled, while the FDA objected to these claims. This pioneering move by Kellogg's in their eighth decade helped pave the way for the Nutrition Labeling and Education Act of 1990 and the Dietary Supplement Health and Education Act of 1994. Despite FDA objections and because there was such a positive response from both consumers and health professionals to the information linking fiber and a decreased risk of colon cancer, legislators were pressured to ensure more health education information on product labels.

Since then, Kellogg's has experimented with psyllium cereal to lower cholesterol levels. They have not been commercially successful, but Quaker has been successful with its oatmeal and oat bran products. Quaker began working with Dr. James Anderson at the University of Kentucky over two decades ago, studying the cholesterol-lowering properties of oatmeal. Over the years, they determined that the soluble portion of oat bran, also called beta glucan, is responsible for lowering cholesterol levels. Recently, Quaker became the first company to receive approval from the FDA for its health claim because the oat-soluble fiber research is so solid. We look at oat bran in more detail in Chapter 9.

CHAPTER 8

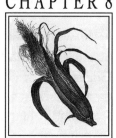

THE BASICS OF INTERNAL CLEANSING

Internal cleansing works in the same way that natural hygiene works on the outside of your body. Your body uses the colon, skin, lungs, and other organs to eliminate toxins as quickly as possible. If these systems are sluggish or over-burdened, the toxins back up into your body and cause headaches, loss of energy, fatigue, aches and pains, and a host of other maladies. Years of improper elimination can lead to the most severe health problems. Internal cleansing is a preventive means to assist your body in keeping its channels of elimination open and clean so that they can perform their vital functions.

The practice of cleansing has existed for thousands of years and has played a central role in the lives of millions of people throughout the world. The Greeks, Romans, Japanese, Turks, Finns, and Russians have all had a form of sauna or bathhouse that played a central role in both their medical practices and social lives. These baths incorporated both sweating and skin brushing as methods to rid the body of stored toxins. The American Indians used their sweat lodges in much the same way. The understanding behind these practices was that cleansing the body of built-up toxins would promote health and prevent degenerative disease. Semiannual trips to the local spa are still a common practice among Europeans.

Dr. Hulda Regehr Clark, author of *The Cure for All Diseases*, points out that all over the world people perform annual cleansing rituals, generally in the spring. In colonial America, people did a sulfur and molasses "cure." In modern America, however, we are lulled into a false sense of security by believing that we are protected from nasty microbes.

Do you need internal cleansing? Look again at the "Autointoxication Checklist" in the Introduction, as well as Figure 8.1, the "Metabolic Screening Questionnaire," and Figure 8.2, the "Dysbiosis Questionnaire and Score Sheet." These tools will help you evaluate your need for some type of internal cleansing program.

In working with patients and training with colleagues, researchers, and scientists over the years, I have developed and promoted several cleansing programs for increasing health and vitality. As I do with my patients and clients, I offer here a number of options to meet your health, time, and budgetary needs. Cleansing products are available in health food stores all over the world; you can purchase and most likely self-administer them safely. Remember, if you are pregnant or have serious health problems, consult first with a health care practitioner before engaging in any cleansing program. It is generally best to work with a trained professional who can support your specific needs, put you in touch with the best products, perform diagnostic

Figure 8.1 Metabolic Screening Questionnaire

Patient Name _____   *Date* _____   *Week* _____

Rate each of the following symptoms
based upon your typical health profile for:
☐ Past 30 days   ☐ Past 48 hours

Point Scale: **0** = *Never or almost never* have the symptom
1 = *Occasionally* have it, effect is *not severe*
2 = *Occasionally* have it, effect is *severe*
3 = *Frequently* have it, effect is *not severe*
4 = *Frequently* have it, effect is *severe*

HEAD	_____ Headaches	
	_____ Faintness	
	_____ Dizziness	
	_____ Insomnia	**Total** _____
EYES	_____ Watery or itchy eyes	
	_____ Swollen, reddened, or sticky eyelids	
	_____ Bags or dark circles under eyes	
	_____ Blurred or tunnel vision (does not include near- or far-sightedness)	**Total** _____
EARS	_____ Itchy ears	
	_____ Earaches, ear infections	
	_____ Drainage from ear	
	_____ Ringing in ears, hearing loss	**Total** _____
NOSE	_____ Stuffy nose	
	_____ Sinus problems	
	_____ Hay fever	
	_____ Sneezing attacks	
	_____ Excessive mucus formation	**Total** _____
MOUTH/ THROAT	_____ Chronic coughing	
	_____ Gagging, frequent need to clear throat	
	_____ Sore throat, hoarseness, loss of voice	
	_____ Swollen or discolored tongue, gums, lips	
	_____ Canker sores	**Total** _____
SKIN	_____ Acne	
	_____ Hives, rash, dry skin	
	_____ Hair loss	
	_____ Flushing, hot flashes	
	_____ Excessive sweating	**Total** _____

Continued

Figure 8.1   (continued)

HEART	_____ Irregular or skipped heartbeat	
	_____ Rapid or pounding heartbeat	
	_____ Chest pain	**Total** _____
LUNGS	_____ Chest congestion	
	_____ Asthma, bronchitis	
	_____ Shortness of breath	
	_____ Difficulty breathing	**Total** _____
DIGESTIVE TRACT	_____ Nausea, vomiting	
	_____ Diarrhea	
	_____ Constipation	
	_____ Bloated feeling	
	_____ Belching, passing gas	
	_____ Heartburn	
	_____ Intestinal/stomach pain	**Total** _____
JOINTS/ MUSCLE	_____ Pain or aches in joint	
	_____ Arthritis	
	_____ Stiffness or limitation of movement	
	_____ Pain or aches in muscles	
	_____ Feeling of weakness or tiredness	**Total** _____
WEIGHT	_____ Binge eating/drinking	
	_____ Craving certain foods	
	_____ Excessive weight	
	_____ Compulsive eating	
	_____ Water retention	
	_____ Underweight	**Total** _____
ENERGY/ ACTIVITY	_____ Fatigue, sluggishness	
	_____ Apathy, lethargy	
	_____ Hyperactivity	
	_____ Restlessness	**Total** _____
MIND	_____ Poor memory	
	_____ Confusion, poor comprehension	
	_____ Poor concentration	
	_____ Poor physical coordination	
	_____ Difficulty in making decisions	
	_____ Stuttering or stammering	
	_____ Slurred speech	
	_____ Learning disabilities	**Total** _____

EMOTIONS	_____	Mood swings	
	_____	Anxiety, fear, nervousness	
	_____	Anger, irritability, aggressiveness	
	_____	Depression	**Total** _____
OTHER	_____	Frequent illness	
	_____	Frequent or urgent urination	
	_____	Genital itch or discharge	**Total** _____
GRAND TOTAL			**TOTAL** _____

Reprinted by permission of HealthComm International, Inc.

work, keep you on track, monitor your progress, and help you through rough spots.

FASTING

Fasting has been used by many cultures as a way of cleansing the body's internal systems. However, fasting can damage the digestive system by starving the microvilli since their preferred food comes from the inside of your gut. Furthermore, during an extended fast you may lose lean body mass, which would cause wasting of your vital organs. Researchers, using rats to discover what effect fasting has on a body, found that the liver has a decreased ability to detoxify pesticides and drugs as early as 36 hours into the fast.

A short fast using pure water and freshly made fruit and/or vegetable juice may allow your body to receive nutrition and avoid starving your digestive lining while giving your system a rest from the work of breaking down large amounts of food into absorbable nutrients. A juice fast, however, may prove harmful to those who are carbohydrate-intolerant. To find out if you are carbohydrate-intolerant, fill out the questionnaire "Determining Your Sensitivity to

Figure 8.2 Dysbiosis Questionnaire and Score Sheet

This questionnaire is designed for adults and the scoring system isn't as appropriate for children. It lists factors in your medical history which are known to contribute to the disruption of normal healthy gastrointestinal bacteria, directly or indirectly promoting the overgrowth of yeasts, fungi, and other pathogens (Section A) and symptoms commonly found in individuals with dysbiosis related illness (Sections B and C).

For each "Yes" answer in Section A, circle the Point Score in that section. Total your score and record it in the box at the end of the section. Then move on to Sections B and C and score as directed.

Filling out and scoring this questionnaire should help you and your physician evaluate the possible role of dysbiosis in contributing to your health problems. Yet it will not provide an automatic "Yes" or "No" answer.

NOTE: Dysbiosis refers to the condition where the normal healthy population of beneficial bacteria in the intestines has been disrupted, leaving it open to the overgrowth of yeast, fungi, parasites, and potentially harmful strains of bacteria. This intestinal imbalance in turn adversely effects other important organ systems via toxic stress and interfering with nutrient absorption and utilization.

Section A: History	Point Score
1. Have you taken tetracyclines (Sumycin, Panmycin, Vibramycin, Minocin, etc.) or other antibiotics for skin, acne, or anything else for 1 month (or longer)?	25
2. Have you, *at any time in your life,* taken other "broad spectrum" antibiotics for respiratory, urinary, or other infections in shorter courses 4 or more times in a 1 year period?	20
3. Have you taken a broad spectrum antibiotic drug— even in a single course?	6
4. Have you, at any time in your life, been bothered by recurrent or persistent prostatitis, vaginitis, or other problems affecting your reproductive organs?	25

5. Have you taken birth control pills . . .

    For more than 5 years?   25

    For more than 2 years?   15

    For 6 months to 2 years?   8

6. Have you been pregnant . . .

    2 or more times?   5

    1 time?   3

7. Have you taken prednisone, Decadron, or other cortisone type drugs . . .

    For more than 6 months?   25

    For more than 2 weeks?   15

    For 2 weeks or less   6

8. Does exposure to perfumes, insecticides, fabric shop odors, and other chemicals provoke . . .

    Moderate to severe symptoms?   20

    Mils symptoms?   5

    List symptoms:

9. Are your symptoms worse on damp, muggy days or in moldy places?   20

    List symptoms:

10. Have you had athlete's foot, ring worm, "jock itch," or other chronic fungous infections of the skin or nails? Y/N

    Have such infections been

        Severe or persistant?   20

        Mild to moderate?   10

11. Do you crave sugar?   10

12. Do you crave breads?   10

13. Do you crave alcoholic beverages?   10

14. Does tobacco smoke really bother you?   10

15. Have you ever had parasitic infection, dysentery, or unexplained episode of prolonged diarrhea and or intestinal distress?   15

Continued

Figure 8.2   (continued)

16. Have you ever consumed chlorinated (or chemically
treated) drinking water for 3 or more months?   15
17. Do you consume commercially raised flesh foods
(antibiotic fed) on a regular basis?   15
18. Do you eat processed foods regularly?   20
19. Do you drink alcohol or consume coffee daily?   20
20. Do you have or have you ever had an ulcer, colitis,
Crohn's disease, or diverticulitis?   35
21. Were you breast fed? If no.   35
If yes, but for less than 3 months.   20

Total Score, Section A   _____

Section B: Major Symptoms   Point Score

For each of your symptoms, enter the appropriate figure in the Point
Score column:
    If a symptom is occasional or mild score 3 pts.
    If a symptom is frequent &/or moderate score 6 pts.
    If a symptom is severe or disabling score 9 pts.
Add total score and record it in the box at the end of this section.

1. Fatigue or lethargy   _____
2. Feeling of being "drained"   _____
3. Poor memory   _____
4. Feeling "spacey" or "unreal"   _____
5. Depression   _____
6. Numbness, burning, or tingling   _____
7. Muscle aches   _____
8. Muscle weakness or paralysis   _____
9. Pain and/or swelling in joints   _____
10. Abdominal pain   _____
11. Constipation   _____
12. Diarrhea   _____
13. Bloating   _____
14. Troublesome vaginal discharge   _____
15. Persistent vaginal burning or itching   _____

16. Prostatitis _____
17. Impotence _____
18. Loss of sexual desire _____
19. Endometriosis _____
20. Cramps and/or other menstrual irregularities _____
21. Premenstrual tension _____
22. Spots in front of eyes _____
23. Erratic vision _____
24. Eczema, dermatitis, psoriasis _____

Total Score, Section B _____

Section C: Other Symptoms   Point Score

For each of your symptoms, enter the appropriate figure in the Point Score column:

    If a symptom is occasional or mild score 3 points.
    If a symptom is frequent and/or moderately severe score 6 points.
    If a symptom is severe and/or disabling score 9 points.

Add total score and record it in the box at the end of this section.

1. Drowsiness _____
2. Irritability or jitteriness _____
3. Incoordination _____
4. Inability to concentrate _____
5. Frequent mood swings _____
6. Headache _____
7. Dizziness/loss of balance _____
8. Pressure above ears . . . feeling of head swelling
   & tingling _____
9. Itching _____
10. Other rashes _____
11. Heartburn _____
12. Indigestion _____
13. Belching and intestinal gas _____
14. Mucus in stools _____

Continued

Figure 8.2   (continued)

15. Hemorrhoids _____
16. Dry mouth _____
17. Rash or blisters in mouth _____
18. Bad breath _____
19. Nasal congestion or discharge _____
20. Joint swelling or arthritis _____
21. Postnasal drip _____
22. Nasal itching _____
23. Sore or dry throat _____
24. Cough _____
25. Pain or tightness in the chest _____
26. Wheezing or shortness of breath _____
27. Urgency or urinary frequency _____
28. Burning on urination _____
29. Failing vision _____
30. Burning or tearing of eyes _____
31. Recurrent infection or fluid in ears _____
32. Ear pain or hearing loss _____

Total Score, Section C _____

Total Score, Section A _____

Total Score, Section B _____

Grand Total Score _____

The Grand Total Score will help you and your physician decide if your health problems are dysbiosis related. Scores in women will run higher as 7 items in the questionnaire apply exclusively to women, while only 2 apply exclusively to men.

Dysbiosis related health problems are almost certainly present in women with scores over 180, and in men with scores over 140.

Dysbiosis related health problems are probably present in women with scores over 120 and in men with scores over 80.

With scores of less than 60 in women and 40 in men, dysbiosis is unlikely to be contributing to your health challenges.

Insulinogenic Foods and Eating Habits." Answer yes or no to each question. The higher your score, the more careful you should be regarding your protein-to-carbohydrate ratio at each meal.

Determining Your Sensitivity to Insulinogenic Foods and Eating Habits

(5) _____ I have a tendency toward high blood pressure.

(5) _____ I gain weight easily, especially around my waist, and I have difficulty losing it.

(5) _____ I often experience mental confusion.

(5) _____ I often experience fatigue and generalized weakness.

(10) _____ I have diabetic tendencies.

(4) _____ I get tired and/or hungry in the mid-afternoon.

(5) _____ About an hour or two after eating a full meal that includes dessert, I want more of the dessert.

(3) _____ It is harder for me to control my eating for the rest of the day if I have a breakfast containing carbohydrates than it would be if I had only coffee or nothing at all.

(4) _____ When I want to lose weight, I find it easier not to eat for most of the day than to try to eat several small diet meals.

(3) _____ Once I start eating sweets, starches, or snack foods, I often have a difficult time stopping.

(3) _____ I would rather have an ordinary meal that included dessert than a gourmet meal that did not include dessert.

(5) _____ After finishing a full meal, I sometimes feel as if I could go back and eat the whole meal again.

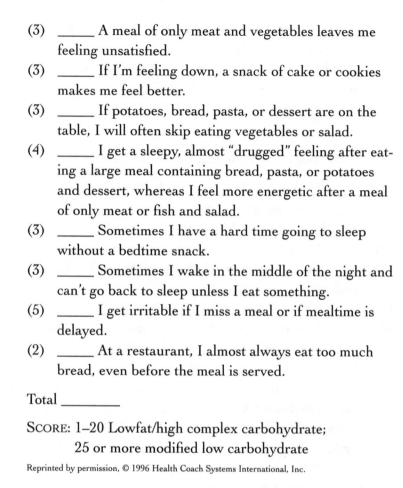

(3) _____ A meal of only meat and vegetables leaves me feeling unsatisfied.

(3) _____ If I'm feeling down, a snack of cake or cookies makes me feel better.

(3) _____ If potatoes, bread, pasta, or dessert are on the table, I will often skip eating vegetables or salad.

(4) _____ I get a sleepy, almost "drugged" feeling after eating a large meal containing bread, pasta, or potatoes and dessert, whereas I feel more energetic after a meal of only meat or fish and salad.

(3) _____ Sometimes I have a hard time going to sleep without a bedtime snack.

(3) _____ Sometimes I wake in the middle of the night and can't go back to sleep unless I eat something.

(5) _____ I get irritable if I miss a meal or if mealtime is delayed.

(2) _____ At a restaurant, I almost always eat too much bread, even before the meal is served.

Total _____

SCORE: 1–20 Lowfat/high complex carbohydrate;
        25 or more modified low carbohydrate

There are studies indicating a need for the amino acid support provided by protein for adequate detoxification of xenobiotics. You may not get the protein you need from a water/juice fast. The "Carbohydrate Classifications of Fruits and Vegetables" chart lists the carbohydrate content of fruits and vegetables. Many people who are carbohydrate-intolerant will find relief from their symptoms just by minimizing grains in their diet without having to consider the carbohydrate content of fruits and vegetables. If that is a factor, which only you can tell through experimentation, it would be wise to choose fruits and vegetables of lower carbohydrate content.

Carbohydrate Classifications of Vegetables
(According to Carbohydrate Content)

3%	6%	15%	20%	25%
Asparagus	Beans, String	Artichokes	Beans, Dried	Potato,
Bean Sprouts	Beets	Carrots	Beans, Lima	Sweet
Beet Greens	Brussels	Oyster Plant	Corn	Yams
Broccoli	Sprouts	Parsnips	Potato, White	
Cabbage	Chives	Peas, Green		
Cauliflower	Collard	Squash		
Celery	Greens			
Chard, Swiss	Dandelion			
Cucumber	Greens			
Endive	Eggplant			
Lettuce	Kale			
Mustard	Kohlrabi			
Greens	Leeks			
Radishes	Onions			
Spinach	Parsley			
Watercress	Peppers, Red			
	Pimento			
	Pumpkin			
	Rutabagas			
	Turnip			

Reprinted by permission Health Coach Systems International, Inc., and New Health Perspectives.

Here are some guidelines for a lower carbohydrate program:

- Eat all of the 3% and 6% vegetable selections that you wish, and the 15% to 25% vegetables in limited quantities. Include only one type of the 15% to 25% vegetables at each meal; they are nutritious and should generally be part of your diet unless your Health Coach has told you otherwise.

- Eat fruit separately from other foods, and preferably in the morning. Choose limited quantities of the 3% or 6% fruit daily, eating a small amount (one cup) at any one time; watch for intolerance to citrus fruit and melons. The 15% to 20% fruits may be selected, but only in small portions at any given time (such as ½ banana or 1 small apple or 3 prunes).

- Eat a large variety of foods, including many different types, but rotate them as much as possible. Avoid eating the same foods day after day.

Carbohydrate Classifications of Fruits (According to Carbohydrate Content)

3 %	6 %	15 %	20 %	25 %
Cantaloupe	Apricots	Apples	Bananas	
Melons	(fresh only)	Blueberries	Figs	
Rhubarb	Blackberries	Cherries	Prunes or any	
Strawberries	Cranberries	Grapes	dried fruits	
Tomatoes	Grapefruit	Kumquats		
Watermelon	Guava	Loganberries		
	Kiwis	Mangoes		
	Lemons	Mulberries		
	Limes	Pears		
	Oranges	Pineapple (fresh)		
	Papayas	Pomegranates		
	Peaches			
	Plums			
	Raspberries			
	Tangerines			

If you lose fat during a fast, you will significantly reduce the toxic load that has accumulated in your body over the years, since most toxins are stored in the fatty tissue in your body. But it's difficult to tell from which of your body tissues you are losing weight by looking in the mirror, trying on tight clothes, or standing on a scale. The weight you lose may be healthy lean tissue if your protein intake is not great enough. During a fast or cleansing program, it is advisable to have your body composition monitored with a bio-impedance system to ensure that you are not losing healthy tissue and that you are instead losing fat and excess water. (Many Health Coaches have this technology in their offices.)

A FOOD ONLY NINE-WEEK CLEANSING PROGRAM

A simple nine-week cleansing program recommended by Health Coach and naturopath Charley Cropley is to eat two servings of fruits, three of vegetables, and one of a whole grain each day for three weeks. During the next three weeks, continue with the fruits, vegetables, and grain and choose, in addition, three consecutive days during the three week period in which you eat only fruits and vegetables. During the last three weeks, continue with the fruit, vegetables, and grain, and choose three consecutive days during which you have only liquids. The liquid diet can consist of fresh fruit and/or vegetable juice and vegetable soup or broth.

Fruits, in general, tend to accelerate cleansing. If your cleansing is going too fast and you are experiencing uncomfortable symptoms, use more vegetables and less fruit. I have included a recipe for Alkaline Broth in Chapter 13 that is nourishing during this three-day cleanse. Some of you may not do well with this program because of the low protein content, but it is simple, inexpensive, and easy to try. During the first three to five days of a cleanse, some people experience symptoms of a cold or flu. If you have these symptoms and they are severe or persist for longer than five days, then consult with your health care practitioner.

Dr. Jeffrey Bland has developed a number of powdered therapeutic food products to support healing of the intestinal tract and detoxification of the liver; they can also help you lose fat and protect against losing protein from your muscles and organs. (For more information on Dr. Bland's detoxification program, see Chapter 10.) These therapeutic foods are available in the offices of licensed health care professionals.

Many Health Coaches have been specially trained to take you through cleansing programs using a modified elimination diet and these healing foods. Any fasting or cleansing program should be monitored carefully, because a drastic cleansing can release toxins too quickly and cause severe reactions.

HERBS

Herbs were the first medicines, and they still provide the ingredients for primary health care in much of the world. Over half of our modern drugs were originally derived from herbs. In my practice, I find that herbs have profound healing abilities without causing many of the insidious side effects of modern synthesized drugs. I utilize chiropractic and herbal healing because both work with the whole person, seeking not only to address specific health complaints but also to accelerate my patients' and clients' progress toward optimal health.

In looking for a good herbal cleansing product, it is most important that the amounts and kinds of herbs interact properly. A formula should be designed so that the herbs work together to promote cleansing and avoid unpleasant reactions. In Chapter 9, I will discuss a program that does just that.

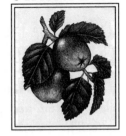

CHAPTER 9

AN HERB
AND FIBER
CLEANSING PROGRAM

Herb and fiber programs have the benefit of cleansing your body without dramatically changing what you are currently eating. This is the preferred method for many people who wish to decrease their toxic burden without making big lifestyle changes. My favorite program in this regard is the Yerba Prima Intestinal Cleansing Program; it is based on ancient traditions of herbal cleansing, yet it suits today's busy lifestyles. I recommend that my patients follow this cleansing program once a year and maintain their colon with a good diet and high-quality fiber supplements between cleansings. The program incorporates herbal formulas in capsule form, called Herbal Guard Caps, Male Rebuild, and Renew and a gentle and effective fiber formula, called Colon Care Formula, which can be purchased in capsule or powder form.

THE YERBA PRIMA INTERNAL CLEANSING PROGRAM

The two requirements for optimum, vibrant health are a clean system and good digestion and assimilation of nutrients. The first step is a clean system. The Internal Cleansing Program supports the elimination organs to more completely remove toxins and waste from the body. It also reduces the reabsorption of toxins from the colon into the bloodstream, protecting against autointoxication. The Internal Cleansing Program promotes regularity in bowel movements and supports healthy liver function—both vital aspects of a healthy digestive system free of toxic buildup. It also helps remove parasites that can live in the body and cause numerous health problems.

REBUILDING DIGESTIVE FUNCTION

The second step toward optimum health is rebuilding the digestive function. Herbs in Herbal Guard Caps, Male Rebuild, and Renew help promote healthy liver, kidney, small intestine, and colon function. They work with Colon Care Formula to promote energy production and rebuilding on a cellular level. They are designed to promote better absorption of nutrients so that you get the most from the foods and supplements you eat. They also support the growth of friendly bacteria and help keep harmful bacteria and yeast populations in balance in your intestines.

The ingredients in the program help the following eliminative and digestive organs and systems: stomach, small intestines, colon, liver, gallbladder, kidneys and urinary system, lymphatic system, respiratory system, skin, and circulatory system. They have the following effects: cleansing, building healthy tissue, anti-oxidant protection, adaptogenic action (helping you to adapt to physical and mental stresses), improving digestion, improving assimilation, carminative action (expelling gas to relieve colic and griping—sharp pains in the bowels), removing parasites, removing toxins, *probiotic* action (promoting the growth of healthy intestinal factors), and renewing energy.

Renew, Male Rebuild, and Herbal Guard Caps

To meet individual needs of men and women, Yerba Prima made Kalenite, the original formula, more gender-specific. For women, they added the nourishing herbs chaste tree berry and dong quai and named the formula "Renew." For men, they added the male support herbs Siberian ginseng and saw palmetto berry and called the formula "Male Rebuild."

Because people are increasingly concerned about the negative effects of foreign and pathogenic microorganisms in their intestines, "Herbal Guard Caps" were developed, drawing upon the wisdom of Western, Native American, Chinese, and Ayurvedic herbalists. The synergistic effects of this herbal formula gently support the detoxification of your digestive system, blood, and lymph while providing nutrients to nourish improved cellular health. If cell health is improved, then so is your total health.

BACKGROUND INFORMATION

A leader in the field of internal cleansing, Yerba Prima sponsored a study in the 1980s to objectively validate the beneficial results reported by people who had used their program, and to contribute to the scientific literature in the area of intestinal health. The study was conducted using the original formulation, Kalenite, along with the Colon Care Formula. The study was designed by Dr. Jeffrey Bland and was performed at the Linus Pauling Institute. The results of the study showed: reduced numbers of pathogenic or harmful bacteria in the colon; significant increase in absorption of water-soluble vitamins; and significant decrease in the putrefaction of undigested protein, indicating better protein absorption by the digestive tract.

Perhaps the most important discovery was that the study subjects felt better after completing the cleanse. They responded with an improved sense of well-being, lower frequency of headaches, and higher energy levels. In fact, they felt so much better that several subjects who had initially been hesitant to begin the cleansing program expressed a desire to use this cleansing program several times a year. The test results showed that the program actively worked to cleanse both the small intestine and the colon. The test subjects were ordinary people who had normal diets and bowel habits and were in good health. They did not shop in health food stores or use herbal products. No dietary changes were requested of them during the study. The study summary said that "even better results" could be expected from this program for people with chronic constipation, poor digestion, prolonged transit times, or low-fiber diets. Generally, "normal" subjects have few effects with health interventions, whereas those who have symptoms or who are ill have pronounced effects.

Yerba Prima has since upgraded the original Kalenite formula to address more current concerns about dysbiosis (see Figure 8.2, Chapter 8)—an overgrowth of pathogenic microbes of all sorts, including bacteria, yeasts, and parasites. The improved formula is the first herbal program I know of that is designed for both complete internal cleansing and rebuilding of good digestion. Because we are exposed to numerous toxins and stresses every day, we need special assistance to maintain good health.

Ingredients of the Intestinal Cleansing Program

Male Rebuild contains: yellow dock root, dandelion leaf and root, Siberian ginseng, red clover, blessed thistle, ginger root, sarsaparilla root, milk thistle seed, plantain leaf, saw palmetto berry, corn silk, and zinc chelate.

Renew (the women's formula) contains: yellow dock root, dandelion leaf and root, red clover, chaste tree berry, ginger root, blessed thistle, dong quai, milk thistle seed, plantain leaf, corn silk, zinc chelate, and the B-vitamins niacinamide, calcium pantothenate, pyridoxine hydrochloride, folic acid, biotin, and cyanocobalamin.

Herbal Guard Caps contain: triphala, elecampane root, ginger root, schisandra berry, cloves, dandelion leaf and root, cat's claw, black walnut hull, and goldenseal root.

Here is a breakdown of the ingredients for Renew and Herbal Guard Caps in alphabetical order:

Black walnut hulls (*Juglans nigra*)   Cleanses: colon
Black walnut hulls are a traditional herb for killing and removing worms and parasites from the body. They also have antifungal properties, including specific effects against candida yeast.

BLESSED THISTLE (*CNICUS BENEDICTUS*)   Cleanses: stomach, liver, gallbladder
Builds: digestion

Blessed thistle has been used for hundreds of years as one of our best mild digestive tonics. Its bitter effect improves digestion and promotes secretion of bile from the liver. Compounds contained within blessed thistle have an antimicrobial effect.

CAT'S CLAW (*UNCARIA TOMENTOSA*)   Cleanses: entire digestive tract and colon
Builds: immune system

Cat's claw, also known as "Una de gato," has been used for hundreds of years by the native people of Peru. It has strong immune-system stimulating properties and promotes the removal of parasites. It also cleanses and heals the entire digestive tract, which helps with many stomach and colon disorders via its anti-inflammatory and anti-oxidant properties.

CHASTE TREE BERRY (*VITEX AGNUS-CASTUS*)   Builds: proper hormonal function

Chaste tree berry is a building and balancing herb for women. It has been used in European herbalism as a tonic and normalizer for the female reproductive system because it helps normalize activity of female sex hormones. This property gives chaste tree berry a wide range of uses, especially in menopause and with any menstrual irregularities. Studies in Europe have shown that this herb helps over time to reduce problems related to PMS.

CLOVES (*SYZYGIUM AROMATICUM*)   Cleanses: colon (antiparasitic), lungs

Builds: digestion

Cloves contain a volatile oil that gives them warming, carminative properties in the stomach and digestive system, which helps to reduce flatulence. It is another synergistic herb in this formula that helps remove worms and parasites from the colon. It is a mild stimulant with expectorant and lung-clearing properties.

CORN SILK (*ZEA MAYS*) Cleanses: kidneys and urinary system

Corn silk has been used for hundreds of years, primarily as a soothing diuretic for the kidneys. It helps reduce inflammation in the urinary system and has a mild cleansing effect on the liver.

DANDELION LEAF AND ROOT (*TARAXACUM OFFICINALE*)
Cleanses: liver, gallbladder, kidneys, blood, skin
Builds: liver and kidney health; nutritive for the entire body

This common weed is used both as food and medicine. We recognize it as an herb for its safe, nutritive, diuretic effect on the kidneys (it is high in potassium) and its ability to stimulate the release of bile and the contraction of the gallbladder, which promotes better bowel movements. David Hoffman, in *Holistic Herbal*, says, "This herb is a most valuable general tonic and perhaps the best widely applicable diuretic and liver tonic." Dandelion has been used for hundreds of years in Europe, the Middle East, China, and India. The first written reference to dandelion as a medicine was from Arabic physicians of the tenth and eleventh centuries A.D. Because it contains polysaccharides, such as inulin, it may provide immune support. It is also known to have anti-inflammatory properties. If dandelion were not such a common plant, and such a pest to the gardener and the grower of manicured lawns, it would probably be hailed as a miracle herb.

As a food, dandelion leaves can be eaten like a vegetable. Tender young leaves add a spark to any salad, and the older, larger leaves are nice to add to sautéed greens for a rich flavor. They are high in vitamins. The roots when roasted have been savored as a coffee substitute.

DONG QUAI ROOT (*ANGELICA SINENSIS*)   Cleanses: blood
Protects: circulatory system, liver
Builds: blood, reproductive system

Dong quai is widely used in Asia, and is considered the premier women's tonic herb. It is used to build the blood and improve circulation. Its other major function is to tonify a woman's reproductive system. For these reasons, it is widely used during menopause as well as throughout the reproductive years.

Dong quai has secondary benefits of protecting the liver, providing mild laxative effects in cases of dry intestines from deficient blood, and contributing antimicrobial properties against many types of bacteria.

ELECAMPANE ROOT (*INULA HELENIUM*)   Cleanses: respiratory system, colon (antiparasitic)
Builds: digestion, general tonic herb

Elecampane root is one of our best antiparasitic herbs. It helps eliminate parasites such as giardia, amebic infections, and pinworms. Even though it is strong, it is safe to use over a long period of time. Traditionally it has been used as a respiratory-system herb, helping to soothe the mucous membranes while clearing and strengthening the lungs and bronchial system. It has mild carminative properties, like ginger and cloves, that soothe digestive upset. Its mild bitter properties improve digestion.

GINGER ROOT (*ZINGIBER OFFICINALE*)   Cleanses: stomach, small intestine, circulatory system, liver
Builds: digestion, stomach, colon, circulatory system

Ginger is *carminative*. Carminative herbs contain essential oils and other constituents that calm the digestive system through their warming, antispasmodic, and anti-inflammatory actions. Cleansing puts stress on the digestive system. Ginger and cloves help to neutralize this stress. Through its anti-inflammatory properties, ginger reduces gas, indigestion, and nausea, as well as having mild pain-relieving effects. It is helpful for motion sickness, and studies show that it is at least as effective as prescription drugs now used for the same purpose without the possible side effects.

Ginger has been used for thousands of years in the Chinese, Ayurvedic, and Western healing traditions, and it tastes good in food or as a stimulating tea that stimulates metabolism. Other beneficial effects include: increased bile secretion; antioxidant protection for the liver; antibacterial properties; anti-parasitic properties (helps eliminate worms); heart protection by lowering cholesterol and inhibiting platelet aggregation; normalization of bowel function; and restoration of colon tone.

GOLDENSEAL ROOT EXTRACT (*HYDRASTIS CANADENSIS*)
Cleanses: digestive system, lungs, reproductive system
Builds: health of mucous membranes, stomach

Goldenseal is widely used among Native Americans, who taught the use of this herb to European settlers. It is one of the best tonic herbs when used in small quantities, as in this formula. In large amounts, it is antimicrobial for mucous membranes of the digestive, respiratory, and reproductive systems. Its bitter quality promotes bile production, improves digestion, and encourages proper bowel movements. Goldenseal has anti-inflammatory, antibacterial, and antiparasitic properties, and is mildly stimulating to the immune system.

MILK THISTLE SEED (*SILYBUM MARIANUM*)   Cleanses: liver, kidneys, blood, skin
Builds: digestion

Milk thistle seed is a mild digestive bitter used in treating skin disorders for its effect on cleansing the blood. Used since antiquity for digestive and liver complaints, it increases secretion and flow of bile. It gently promotes liver cleansing, but its primary actions go beyond that as one of the strongest liver herbs known. It both protects the liver with its anti-oxidant properties and rebuilds by supporting RNA synthesis.

The toxins our liver neutralizes come from within us as well as from the outside world. During the cleansing process, the liver has extra work to do as toxins are released from tissues of the body into the blood and lymph. Milk thistle seed extract protects the liver cells as they neutralize toxins, bind to them, and dump them into the colon for elimination from the body. At the same time, milk thistle seed extract is working to rebuild damaged liver tissue.

The primary activity of this herb is due to compounds in the seeds known as *silymarin*, a group of *flavnolignan* (a large class of substances found in plants that have healing properties) compounds, which have been studied extensively for the past few decades, primarily in Europe. Silymarin has been used successfully to treat patients who have chronic hepatitis and cirrhosis; it is active against hepatitis-B virus, and it lowers fat deposits in the liver in animals.

Historical use of milk thistle as a liver herb dates back to the first century. Pliny the Elder, a Roman naturalist, tells us that the juice of the plant mixed with honey is excellent for "carrying off bile." Bile is a concentrated liver product that is excreted from the gallbladder in response to dietary fats in the small intestines.

Recently, European doctors have found that they can save the lives of most people who would have died from mistakenly eating the poisonous *Amanita phalloides* mushroom ("death cap"). They do this by intravenous drip injection with a pure extract of milk thistle seed called "Silibinin" within forty-eight hours of exposure. Prior to this discovery, about twenty-five percent of the unfortunate mushroom hunters died from hemorrhagic necrosis of the liver, or they had to undergo liver transplant surgery with subsequent immunosuppressive therapy for the rest of their lives to help them tolerate the new organ.

Because of its effect on cleansing the blood, milk thistle is also used for treating skin disorders.

PLANTAIN LEAF (*PLANTAGO MAJOR* OR *PLANTAGO LANCEO-LATA*)   Cleanses: kidneys and urinary system, respiratory system, colon

Plantain leaf is a soothing herb with mild diuretic, expectorant, and digestion-enhancing properties. It is an excellent supportive herb for the cleansing process. Plantain contains mucilage, which provides soothing action and helps heal inflamed tissue in the colon and rectum. Plantain leaf juice and syrups have been used in Europe to reduce symptoms of bronchitis and respiratory problems. It has mild liver-cleansing and bowel-regulating properties, and acts as a mild antimicrobial.

RED CLOVER TOPS (*TRIFOLIUM PRATENSE*)   Cleanses: blood, liver, lymphatic system
Builds: blood
Although there is not a lot of clinical research, red clover has a long history of use as a general cleansing and building herb. During colds it has been used to calm coughs (antispasmodic) and to promote the ejection of mucus and other fluids from the upper respiratory tract. It has soothing and relaxing properties, while supporting lymphatic activity.

SARSAPARILLA ROOT (*SMILAX SPP.*)   Cleanses: blood
Protects: liver, colon
Builds: energy levels, blood
Sarsaparilla root is not just an ingredient in soft drinks. It is a tonic and a building herb used in many cultures around the world for its gentle strengthening properties. More recently, it has been widely used by athletes to support the muscle-building and strengthening process.

Traditionally, sarsaparilla root has been used to treat rheumatism and skin conditions in both Europe and Asia. It works through the liver and kidneys to cleanse and build the blood. In addition, it contributes mild anti-inflammatory properties.

SAW PALMETTO BERRY (*SERENOA REPENS*)   Protects: prostate
Builds: general nutritional support
Saw palmetto berry helps strengthen the male reproductive system. It is best known for its ability to protect and

support proper functioning of the prostate gland. This has been proven in numerous double-blind studies in Europe, even when compared with prescription drugs used to treat benign prostatic hypertrophy. Traditionally, saw palmetto berry has been used by Native Americans as a nutritive tonic.

SCHISANDRA BERRY (*SCHISANDRA CHINENSIS*)   Cleanses: liver
Builds: liver, energy, digestion, adrenal glands

In your liver, the adaptogen schisandra offers strong liver protection; it is an anti-oxidant that promotes repair of damaged liver tissue. It promotes better digestion, builds kidney function, and normalizes stomach acidity. Through its mild stimulating effect on the central nervous system, it promotes energy gently while increasing stamina and endurance. Studies have shown that schisandra has the ability to quicken reflexes and improve a person's ability to perform concentrated work.

SIBERIAN GINSENG ROOT (*ELEUTHEROCOCCUS SENTICOSUS*)
Protects: immune system
Builds: adrenal glands, energy levels

Siberian ginseng root is one of the primary *adaptogenic* herbs, meaning that it helps a person adapt to physical and psychological stressors. It is a building herb that is safe to use on a daily basis. It helps build energy without stimulating, and reduces the harmful effects of stress on the body. Siberian ginseng root helps protect and build both the adrenal glands and the immune system.

Since the 1960s, hundreds of studies have been published in Russia on the beneficial effects of Siberian ginseng, and now it is used worldwide.

TRIPHALA (A COMBINATION OF THREE HERBS: *PHYLLAN-THUS EMBLICA, TERMINALIA BALLERICA, TERMINALIA CHEBULA*)

Cleanses: stomach, small intestine, colon, respiratory system
Builds: stomach, small intestine, colon, overall digestion

This herb combination comes to us from Ayurveda, the ancient East Indian tradition of healing. Traditionally, triphala has been used as a bowel normalizer for either constipation or diarrhea and to improve the tone of the colon through the astringent properties of tannins. Triphala helps purify the blood through its actions against bacteria, yeast, fungus, parasites, and worms. It promotes normal appetite and good digestion, while improving the absorption of B-vitamins. Like ginseng in Asia, triphala is used as an adaptogen and a rejuvenating food in the Ayurvedic system of health care. It has been found to be of special value both as a regulator of elimination and a revitalizer of the entire body.

YELLOW DOCK ROOT (*RUMEX CRISPUS*)   Cleanses: liver, gallbladder, colon, blood, lymph, respiratory system, skin
Builds: liver, blood, digestive system

Yellow dock root supports the function of the liver and gall bladder by promoting bile secretion and flow, which indirectly supports the colon with a gentle laxative action. Throughout history, *bitters* such as yellow dock root have been used to stimulate appetite and digestion. Bitters are herbs that activate gastric secretion of hydrochloric acid and other digestive enzymes such as bile. Another historical use of this herb, which goes back thousands of years, is for cleansing. It was widely used by almost twenty Native American tribes. Through its antibacterial properties, it improves skin conditions. Yellow dock root is also high in iron and promotes better use of iron in the body. It has a gentle effect over time that helps promote regular elimination.

THE COLON CARE FORMULA

To complement the herbal activity of Herbal Guard Caps, Renew, and Male Rebuild, Yerba Prima developed a high-fiber formula called the "Colon Care Formula" as an essential part of the cleansing program. (See Chapters 3 and 7 for information on the importance of dietary fiber.) Mixed fiber products show the best anticancer effects. This formula is made from a variety of fiber sources, plus other protective nutrients, and is designed to perform the following functions:

- Absorb the toxins that are being released by the body into the colon (animal studies indicate that various drugs, chemicals, and food additives are highly toxic when fed to rats and mice in conjunction with a purified, low-fiber diet; when fed diets high in dietary fiber, the same doses have no deleterious effects).
- Speed the toxic-laden feces out of the body rapidly and regularly.
- Promote stools that are larger, softer, and easier to evacuate.
- Reduce pressure in the colon and lessen the risk of diverticulosis, hemorrhoids, and other colon disorders.
- Help build the population of friendly bacteria in the intestines, thus encouraging a strong and toxic-free system.

- Provide "food" to the colon's friendly bacteria
  to enhance the production of B-vitamins, mammalian lignans, and SCFAs (short chain fatty
  acids) which are a by-product of friendly intestinal
  bacteria which act as a nutrient source for cells
  lining the intestinal tract (this in turn protects
  against cancer and helps to maintain the integrity
  of the colon lining).
- Increase absorption of nutrients across the bowel
  wall.
- Decrease the risk of colon, breast, and prostate
  cancer.
- Decrease the risk of heart disease.

The ingredients in Colon Care Formula work together to achieve optimal benefits (see pages 151–153 for
usage). Colon Care Formula and Colon Care Caps contain
the following fibers and colon-nourishing supplements: psyllium seed husks, calcium carbonate, FOS probiotic growth
complex (fructooligosaccharides), acacia gum, barley bran,
oat bran, and fruit pectin.

PSYLLIUM SEED HUSKS   Cleanses: intestinal tract
Protects: colon and circulatory systems (cholesterol lowering)
Builds: colon cells
    Psyllium was first introduced as a commercial product
in the United States, not by health food stores but by the
Kellogg brothers, according to the Director of Research at
Kellogg's. John Harvey Kellogg found psyllium on a trip to
Sicily and introduced it at the Battle Creek Sanitarium.
Beginning in the 1920s, it was sold at the sanitarium under
the name "Psylla." After the sanitarium folded, psyllium was

forgotten by Kellogg's until the late 1980s. At that time, Kellogg's scientists were seeing research that soluble fiber helped lower cholesterol levels and reduce the risk of heart disease. Kellogg's had found great sales success with their educational campaign telling people how fiber could reduce the risk of cancer. They saw the possibility for similar success with a soluble-fiber cereal. So Kellogg's scientists tested 100 different sources of soluble fibers and decided that psyllium was the best of all. Psyllium husk is highly concentrated in its activity and retains its effectiveness even after processing into a breakfast cereal. But Kellogg's psyllium-based cereals have not met sales expectations in the United States, and the name "Heartwise" was discontinued. However, they have a better-selling psyllium cereal in Australia being marketed for heart health.

For health and cleansing, psyllium husk can be considered the best choice. As we shall see, though, other fiber sources have important benefits. Psyllium is the most exciting because of its broad range of cleansing actions in the body. It has the properties of both soluble and insoluble fibers. In general, insoluble fibers add bulk and attract water into your bowel; whereas soluble fibers are responsible for the other heart-healthy, cancer-protective, bacteria-building properties. Psyllium fiber both adds bulk, acting as a gentle broom for your intestinal lining, and lowers cholesterol levels to protect your cardiovascular system against heart attacks.

No cleansing program can be successful without removing toxins from the colon, and studies have shown that no fiber is as powerful as psyllium husks for trapping and removing toxins. Imagine a sponge that expands forty to seventy times its original size, with expanded scrubbing power. That gives you a picture of the power of psyllium. Psyllium husks form a soft, bulky mass that gently scrubs the walls of the intestines as it moves through your digestive tract. At the same time, it traps toxins and excess cholesterol and flushes them out of your body.

Psyllium contributes to the cleansing process in a multitude of ways. In addition to scrubbing the colon walls and removing toxins, it promotes a shorter transit time. This means that the body's waste material spends less time in your colon and has less contact with the mucosa of your colon.

Psyllium husks strengthen the integrity of the intestinal lining, reducing the chance of bacteria and intestinal toxins penetrating through the wall and into your blood stream. Animal studies showed that adding fiber to a liquid diet reduced the amount of bacteria crossing the intestinal wall and getting into the circulation by almost 90 percent. This may be accomplished through the nourishment SCFAs provide to the cells lining the intestines. As one of the soluble fibers, psyllium husks promote the growth of friendly bacteria in the colon. Friendly bacteria support the cleansing process and help restore normal bowel function.

CALCIUM CARBONATE   Cleanses: colon
Builds: bones, circulatory system, holds cells together

Colon cancer is the second most common cancer in women and the third most common in men. Animals and people who eat a high-fat, low-fiber diet get colon cancer more often. When animals are injected with carcinogenic substances, those fed high-fat diets have a higher incidence of cancer than those fed lowfat diets. Calcium is protective against colon cancer. It works through several different modes of action. Supplementing dietary calcium at about 1.5 times the Recommended Dietary Allowance (for a total of 1,500 milligrams/day) restores the cells of your colon wall to a more normal and quiet equilibrium, reducing the over-proliferation that occurs with cancer growth. And calcium that is not absorbed by the small intestine enters the colon and binds with rancid fats and excess bile acids to form harmless insoluble soaps. The protective properties of calcium complement the protective properties of insoluble fiber.

High phosphate levels in the diet, from soda and carbonated beverages, will cause phosphate to bind with calcium and reduce its ability to remove rancid fats, toxins, and excess bile acids from the colon.

FOS Probiotic Growth Complex (also known as: Fructooligosaccharides)   Cleanses: colon
Builds: colon cells, friendly intestinal bacteria

Fructooligosaccharides (FOS) are naturally occurring complex sugars that have beneficial effects in your diet. They can be found in rye, banana, onion, garlic, burdock, asparagus, chicory root, and Jerusalem artichoke. Judging from usual eating habits, it may be difficult to ingest the recommended daily doses of FOS from foods. Most animal and human diets are deficient in FOS.

In addition, most modern people engage in activities that cause damage to their intestines: overconsumption of alcohol; eating raw eggs, fish, and seafood that may produce bacterial infections; use of aspirin and other pain killers; use of antibiotics; and poor diet. Every year over thirty-five million pounds of antibiotics are consumed by humans, livestock, and poultry in the United States. You may unknowingly consume second-hand antibiotics hidden in meat, poultry, and dairy products unless you eat organic animal products raised without the use of antibiotics. The overall effect of our antibiotic habit has not only been the destruction of helpful bacteria in the intestines but also the establishment of harmful strains of bacteria that antibiotics can no longer kill.

Over the last thirty years of antibiotic use, strains of bacteria have mutated to become antibiotic-resistant for almost every known bacterial disease. In 1992, 13,300 hospital patients died of infections that resisted every drug their doctor tried, and in 1993 the number grew to 70,000. Dr. Bill Jarvis of the Centers for Disease Control and Prevention in Atlanta said, "[Resistance to antibiotics] is probably the number-one public health issue."

Unless you are eating a significant quantity of foods high in FOS, you would benefit from the addition of FOS products to your daily regimen such as Colon Care Formula from Yerba Prima or Ultra Flora Plus and Probioplex Intensive Care from Metagenics (see Appendix 1 for more information). Extensive animal and human studies have established the safety and efficacy of FOS. It is now used as an ingredient in over five hundred food products in Japan. In studies done with FOS, stool markers (laboratory stool tests) dropped down to less healthy levels when FOS was withdrawn from the diet. Health contributions of FOS arise from its unique fermentation characteristics:

FOS increases the population of bifidobacteria (*bifs*) and lactobacilli in your colon even without adding probiotic cultures to your diet. The FOS-nourished bifs decrease stool pH, which inhibits the growth of undesirable organisms and stimulates your gut's immune system, perhaps due to an increased production of SCFAs. By suppressing the activity of undesirable putrefactive bacteria, such as *E. coli, Salmonella,* and *Clostridium perfringens,* bifs reduce the formation of their toxic fermentation products.

This in turn protects your liver function by reducing levels of toxic bowel metabolites. Your liver is saved from having to process these harmful by-products of a low-fiber, high-fat diet and poor digestion.

People with diarrhea and soft, loose stools found that their bowel movements shifted to a firmer consistency and that constipation was prevented through production of SCFAs, which stimulate bowel motility (peristalsis) and increase fecal moisture and osmotic pressure.

Sustained intake of FOS among the Japanese in the mid-1980s resulted in significant reductions in cholesterol and triglyceride levels, just like adding additional fiber. Fiber and FOS have a synergistic effect. FOS also caused a reduction of blood pressure; the more bifs present, the lower the *diastolic* blood pressure (the bottom number, which indicates the pressure in your heart).

FOS has an anticancer effect due to immunity enhancements by the cells, cell wall components, and extracellular components of bifidobacteria.

Finally, FOS supports production of the vitamins B_1, B_2, B_3, B_6, B_{12}, and folic acid. These are all part of the B-complex vitamins, which support your brain, nervous system, digestion, and energy production.

ACACIA GUM   Builds: intestinal tract by feeding healthy bacteria and intestinal cells

Acacia gum is a concentrated source of soluble fiber. Unlike most soluble fibers, it does not form thick solutions when mixed with water. Acacia gum is totally broken down as a food source for beneficial intestinal bacteria, such as bifs and other friendly bacteria increasing their numbers in your colon. With the increase in bacterial mass, it also slightly increases the bulk material in the colon. However, it does not improve transit time as do psyllium husks and barley bran.

Acacia gum has been shown to slightly reduce elevated cholesterol levels. Its effect is not as strong as that of psyllium husks, oat bran, and pectin. In human trials, the addition of acacia gum to a glucose (sugar) load resulted in significant reduction of sugar and insulin in the blood when taken at the same time. It acts as a *demulcent,* or soothing substance, for the lining of the intestinal tract. Acacia gum is widely used in foods such as beverages, salad dressings, and sauces as a carrier for flavors and as a stabilizer. Like FOS, though to a lesser extent, acacia gum protects colon cells against cancer by increasing their depth; the cell actually becomes deeper, thus tonifying the bowel. (Cells are supposed to be deep; when they are not, it is a sign of cancer.)

BARLEY BRAN   Cleanses: colon
Builds: healthy bacteria

Barley bran contains a variety of nutrients, including insoluble fiber, to feed healthy bacteria. It has been a food source for thousands of years and was one of the first cereal grains that was farmed. Barley was the primary grain used for making bread in medieval Europe, but it is now grown primarily as animal feed and for brewing beer. It is high in insoluble fiber. This kind of fiber helps keep you regular and protects against the risk of colon cancer. Insoluble fibers shorten transit time, which means that waste material moves through the colon more quickly, leaving less time for toxins to be in contact with the intestinal lining and reducing the chance that the toxins will be reabsorbed into the bloodstream through the colon. Barley bran dilutes the contents of the feces through its bulking action.

Researchers in Denmark, Norway, and England found that study subjects who ate barley bran reported decreased hunger feelings compared to non-fiber-supplemented controls. In another study, taking barley bran led to significant weight loss over a year every time weight was measured at eleven, sixteen, and fifty-two weeks.

Research in the United States shows that a combination of psyllium husks and wheat bran is more protective against colon cancer than wheat bran alone. Work in Australia indicates that barley bran may provide even stronger protection against colon cancer than wheat bran. Thus, a combination of fibers such as psyllium husks, barley bran, and others is ideal not only for cleansing your system but also for protecting you against the development of colon cancer.

OAT BRAN   Cleanses: colon; lowers elevated cholesterol and triglyceride levels
Builds: health of circulatory system; high in nutrients for whole body

Dozens of studies have consistently shown that oat bran consumption causes a significant reduction in elevated cholesterol and triglyceride levels. The soluble-fiber portion of oat bran is believed to be responsible for this benefit. About half of the fiber in oat bran is soluble fiber. In this way, the humble oat can help reduce the risk of heart diseases at the same time that it provides nutrition.

Oat bran should not be confused with fiber from the hull of the oat, sometimes called "oat fiber." The hull is removed before oats are used for human food, and it is entirely insoluble fiber. It does not have the cholesterol-lowering properties of oat bran, and some unscrupulous companies sell it because it costs less than oat bran.

FRUIT PECTIN   Cleanses: intestinal tract, circulatory system (cholesterol and blood glucose lowering)
Builds: colon health

Pectin is a soluble fiber that is found in all fruits and vegetables, but especially in apples and citrus fruit. It has a number of beneficial properties in the body. Pectin lowers elevated cholesterol levels, as do many soluble fibers. However, other properties of pectin are actually more important.

Pectin is almost entirely fermented by intestinal bacteria, which means that it is used as a food source by the "good guys" in your intestines. As you have previously read, these friendly bacteria synthesize B-vitamins, acidify the colon, produce SCFAs, protect the colon, and keep harmful bacteria and yeasts in check.

Pectin consumed with meals increases excretion of fecal fat, neutral steroids, and fecal bile acids. By increasing the excretion of fecal neutral steroids, it helps reduce your risk of sex-hormone-related cancers. Remember that old adage, "An apple a day keeps the doctor away." Apples are high in pectin, ridding your body of excess cancer-stimulating hormones.

The addition of pectin to a drink or meal significantly reduces blood glucose response. The inclusion of pectin in the diets of diabetics would be beneficial in the treatment of diabetes. However, this effect is dependent on the presence of pectin in the intestine during the sugar stress. The sugar-stabilizing effect is also felt by normal subjects, helping to diminish blood sugar swings and drastic changes in mood and energy.

The feeding of pectin, unlike other fiber sources such as wheat bran, does not decrease the level of minerals, such as calcium, magnesium, zinc, and copper, in the blood. However, iron levels have been shown to be decreased by pectin in some but not all human studies.

Pectin is also known to pick up heavy metals as it goes through the digestive tract. Russian research showed that pectin and pectin-containing foods increased the excretion of lead, mercury, manganese, and beryllium from the gastrointestinal tract. It also protected animals and people from lead poisoning when taken before and during exposure to lead.

USAGE INSTRUCTIONS

Although each person's needs will vary, in this section I will provide general guidelines for following a detoxification program with the Yerba Prima Herb and Fiber Cleansing Program. Consult your health care practitioner before beginning any detoxification program. If problems arise, stop using the products and consult with your health care practitioner. Pregnant and lactating women should not engage in detoxification.

As indicated on the package, for the first three to seven days (level one), take one capsule each of Herbal Guard Caps and Renew or Male Rebuild with four capsules

Recommended Amounts for Colon Care Products

Women

Time Period	Herbal Guard Caps	Renew	Colon Care Formula
3 to 7 days	1	1	4
2 to 8 weeks	2	2	6

Men

Time Period	Herbal Guard Caps	Male Rebuild	Colon Care Formula
3 to 7 days	1	1	4
2 to 8 weeks	2	2	6

of Colon Care Formula and a minimum of eight ounces of pure water. For the next five to seven weeks, take two each of Herbal Guard Caps and the Renew or Male Rebuild with six capsules of Colon Care Formula and a minimum of eight ounces of pure water. (See Chapters 3 and 7 for more information about fiber in your diet.) The chart above gives the indications for usage.

If you find ongoing benefit from taking the herbal formulas, you can continue to take them in conjunction with the Colon Care products for longer than eight weeks. For those with a low-fiber diet, regular use of Colon Care Formula or caps would greatly support your health.

You will benefit from this cleansing program with almost any kind of diet. However, chances are you will increase your benefits significantly by following these daily guidelines: eat five servings of fruits and vegetables and drink sufficient pure water (for your body weight, see pages 193–194) to aid detoxification.

Keeping a diary to chart your progress will aid your appreciation of the necessity and benefit of engaging in regular detoxification programs. The "Bowel Movement Progress Chart," page 170, can assist your progress toward vibrant good health.

CHAPTER 10

THERAPEUTIC FOOD POWDERS FOR CLEANSING

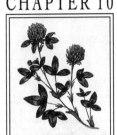

Cleansing programs that use therapeutic food powders spare protein loss and provide specific nutrition for the support and repair of organ systems during detoxification. Dr. Jeffrey Bland has developed a line of therapeutic food powders that are effective for cleansing the body and supporting your inherent ability to heal. The therapeutic foods are tasty and easy to use. I personally use these products almost daily, and for regular cleansing programs several times per year. It's easy to get good nutrition with this Ultra line of products. They are reasonably priced, and they beat chopping, cooking, and cleaning up after yourself when you have limited time. Many of my patients and clients, as do I, choose to have an Ultra drink for breakfast. Since the food powders are made of small food molecules, they are easy to digest and absorb when you are in a rush to eat before or during your work day. The cleansing Ultra products—Ultra Clear, Ultra Clear Plus, and Ultra Clear Sustain—are available only through offices of licensed health care practitioners. Cleansing programs using these products must be performed in conjunction with a health care practitioner who can determine the specifics regarding quantity, dosage, frequency, length of the cleanse, and the most appropriate food powder to use.

Dr. Bland and a group of registered dietitians, scientists, and medical doctors conducted studies using these products. In order to assess the need for cleansing and chart the progress of the subjects tested, several tools were used, including the Metabolic Screening Questionnaire (MSQ) in Chapter 8 and a liver function test called the Functional Liver Detoxification Profile (FLDP), which measured the breakdown products of caffeine and sodium benzoate in saliva and urine. The FLDP measures the detoxification processes of the liver. These tests differ from the normal liver blood tests in that the FLDP measures the ability of the liver to do its job, whereas normal blood tests measure the enzymes from dying (necrosing) liver tissue.

The FLDP is a measure of how your body detoxifies commonly used liver stressors: caffeine, acetaminophen, and aspirin. Caffeine is converted into a benign substance through a process in the liver called the "phase I cytochrome P450 mixed oxidase pathway." Aspirin and acetaminophen are metabolized through both the "phase I and phase II pathways." Phase I detoxification is stimulated through exposure to xenobiotics, steroids, toxics produced inside the body, alcohol, and chemical substances. If you are the kind of person who has a marked reaction to caffeine that lasts for hours and interferes with your ability to sleep even though you may have had it early in the day, then you probably have suppressed phase I detoxification in your liver.

(Remember Tom Latimer in Chapter 5? His phase I detoxification was suppressed by the medication Tagamet.) Phase I detoxification converts toxics and normal chemical substances such as hormones into intermediary metabolites; these are often more dangerous and carcinogenic than the chemicals to which a person was initially exposed. That is why you need a well-functioning phase II: to complete the job of phase I and make those toxic intermediary metabolites into benign end-products that can be safely eliminated from your body, primarily through secretion into your blood and subsequent excretion in urine through your kidneys, but also through secretion into the bile and subsequent excretion in the feces.

Have you or someone you know experienced a "cleansing reaction" when you were attempting to detoxify your body? What's happening in this situation is that phase I detoxification has been stimulated, or upregulated, without having the support of ample nutrients to complete the process through phase II into harmless products. The intermediary metabolites instead reenter your bloodstream and wreak havoc among your many cells and body systems. If you are a "canary" with multiple food and chemical sensitivities who is bothered by the smell of perfume and car fumes, especially diesel exhaust (perfumes are often derivatives of petroleum), you probably have too little phase II conjugates to detoxify the intermediary metabolites produced by phase I in your liver.

What Dr. Bland's team of researchers found was amazing. In a study of normal, nondiseased, but unwell people, published in *The Journal of Applied Nutrition* (vol. 44, no. 3&4, 1992) doctors Bland and Bralley found that the chronic symptoms in the group that was using Ultra Clear were much lower in intensity, duration, and frequency than among those on the placebo diet. The greatest improvements occurred with "tired eyes" and "pain behind the eyes," headaches, gastrointestinal disturbances, morning pain and stiffness, and chronic respiratory complaints. The therapeutic food group's objective laboratory test results improved more than the placebo diet group. The MSQ scores for the test diet group lowered significantly; scores for the placebo group did not. Both phases of liver detoxification for the test group worked better; the placebo group did not improve significantly. The study report states: "These data suggest a relationship between improved liver detoxification and decreased chronic symptoms and health complaints in non-diseased people." The therapeutic food group gained better health in only twenty-one days.

AN EFFECTIVE CLEANSING PROGRAM FOR OVERCOMING CHRONIC FATIGUE

Chronic Fatigue Immunodeficiency Syndrome (CFIDS) is thought to be caused by a viral agent. A study titled, "Management of Chronic Fatigue Symptoms by Tailored Nutrition Using a Program Designed to Support Hepatic Detoxification," by doctors Rigden, Bralley, and Bland shows that, for some, the signs and symptoms of CFIDS can be relieved by supporting liver detoxification. Perhaps you don't fit the Center for Disease Control's criteria for CFIDS (pages 161–162), but chances are that you feel drained sometimes. Maybe that second wind just won't seem to kick in even with your usual remedies and stimulants. Fatigue is the most common symptom that patients report to their doctor.

Doctors Rigden, Bralley, and Bland documented the health improvements in thirty patients who fulfilled the Center for Disease Control's criteria for CFIDS. The average time these subjects had suffered with CFIDS symptoms before participating in this study was three years, and they had all tried many other therapies to regain their health before trying Dr. Bland's therapeutic food, Ultra Clear. After only seven days of following the nutritional intervention program based on Ultra Clear, the test subjects showed marked improvement in eye, respiratory, central nervous system, and musculoskeletal symptoms. Whereas the Metabolic Screening Questionnaire mean score for the nondiseased people was 44, the average score among the CFIDS participants was 173. That score dropped in half after only one month of nutritional intervention. The most significant reduction of symptoms was associated with improvements in vision-related problems (tired eyes and inability to read for any length of time). Other improvements included a reduction of headaches, improvements in respiratory function, reduced sinusitis and congestion, and improvements in central nervous system function.

One participant, who had been unable to work for a year, was back at work and functioning well with her family responsibilities after the nutritional intervention program. Another participant was an accountant who, due to the symptoms of CFIDS, had become unable to work with numbers. After the cleansing program, which reduced her symptoms by more than fifty percent, she was able to return to work. The clinical improvement in the symptoms and abnormalities found in the immune systems of people with CFIDS were closely related to improved activity of both phase I and II of liver detoxification in functional lab tests.

They enjoyed these beneficial results from doing cleansing programs using the Ultra Clear products under the supervision of a health care practitioner.

Dr. Jeffrey Bland and his team evaluated the effectiveness of the therapeutic food supplement Ultra Clear Sustain (UCS) for detoxification versus a hypoallergenic, calorie-controlled diet alone in the management of chronically ill patients. There were 106 patients chosen for the study. The eighty-four patients in the experimental group who consumed the UCS had a fifty-two-percent reduction in symptoms over ten weeks using the Metabolic Screening Questionnaire (MSQ) on pages 111–113. The twenty-two patients on the control diet had only a twenty-two percent reduction of symptoms. In the group that used UCS, symptoms reduced and the Functional Liver Detoxification Profile (FLDP) showed normalization of both phases of liver detoxification. Enhanced nutrient absorption was implied by positive results in bowel function tests.

The patients in this study were free of serious disease. However, they suffered with fatigue, muscle and joint pain, chronic gastrointestinal problems, headaches, sleep disturbances, and cognitive impairment (which the patients often described as "brain fog") of at least one year's duration (average 2.4 years). Patients in both groups were placed on food-elimination diets to reduce their intake of the most common allergens: dairy products, gluten-containing grains, and citrus fruits. They were also asked to avoid red meat, pork, veal, and all products containing alcohol and caffeine, including over-the-counter medications.

Symptoms that improved most rapidly were those related to energy/activity, digestive functions, mood/mind/

emotions, sleep, and muscle pain. Additional symptoms that improved were those related to eye pain when reading, headaches, and skin problems. In a subgroup of the therapeutic food patients who had GI disturbances, symptoms such as flatulence, bloating, alternating constipation and diarrhea, and intestinal pain after eating were reduced after intervention. Although the control group on the food program alone showed improvement in the MSQ, no significant changes were measured in their objective lab tests.

It becomes obvious from these studies that the best way to treat your body during a cleanse is to give it nourishing, easy-to-digest foods or food powders to enhance your body's ability to heal. There are many food powders on the market. To make sure you are investing in a product that supports your health, it is best to read the ingredient list carefully. If the product has anything artificial in it, I would recommend finding another product. The same goes for sugar (sucrose, dextrose), NutraSweet (aspartame), Sweet 'n Low (saccharine), and other sweeteners. A food powder to avoid is the popular Ultra Slim Fast that is sold in many supermarkets. It has been shown to help people lose weight, but most of the weight lost is lean weight from muscles, organs, and glands, not fat. This compromises both your health and longevity and works against your liver's ability to cleanse toxins from your body.

Chronic Fatigue Syndrome Questionnaire

1. I have experienced easy fatigability that has lasted at least six months.

2. A physician has evaluated me and ruled out any physical or psychiatric diseases that may mimic CFS symptoms.
3. For at least the past six months, I have experienced recurring or persisting:
   a. chills or mild fever; rash over one year that comes and goes
   b. sore throats
   c. painful or swollen lymph glands
   d. unexplained general muscle weakness
   e. fatigue for 24 hours after previously tolerated exercise
   f. headaches unlike any previously experienced
   g. joint pain without joint swelling or redness
   h. forgetfulness
   i. excessive irritability
   j. confusion
   k. inability to concentrate
   l. depression
   m. disturbed sleep

If you answered yes to questions one and two and marked at least eight of the criteria in question 3, then you may have CFS.

Criteria developed by The Centers for Disease Control and Prevention.

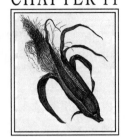

CHAPTER 11

CLEANSING THE LIVER AND THE LYMPH SYSTEM

CLEANSING THE LIVER

In addition to the other recommendations I have made for cleansing, a good liver cleanse is of great benefit. It is easiest on your body to do a liver flush after completing a program that addresses your colon health. If you attempt to do a liver cleanse when you have a toxic bowel, you will be dumping toxic contents from your liver into an already toxic environment. Under these circumstances you are virtually guaranteed to get sick from liver detoxification.

If you cleanse your colon first, you cut down on the waste and toxins that your liver has to deal with; your liver gets a break so it has an opportunity to heal better on its own.

Our livers have an amazing capacity to heal. If eighty percent of your liver is destroyed, it will grow back and work for you again. This may have something to do with the abundant amount of blood delivered to this vital organ of detoxification. Your liver gets twenty percent of your blood supply, even though it weighs only about four pounds

Dietary Changes to Cleanse the Liver

What you put into your mouth is number one. Fried and greasy foods are challenging for your liver to process, especially because of the damaging qualities of most of the commercially available fats and oils. Alcohol is another substance that commands a lot of attention from your liver. Eliminating those two classes of food and beverage stress will give your liver a break and allow it to begin the process of repair. Also, you would benefit by eliminating or minimizing refined carbohydrates from your diet, such as sugar, white bread, rolls and pasta, and pastries, cakes, and cookies.

Eating foods and herbs that are nourishing for your liver is the next step. The green leafy tops of beets are one of the best foods for your liver. You can steam them just like spinach, and put a little lemon on them if you like. They're healthy and delicious. Or you can put the small young leaves in a salad for a new taste sensation and a little added color. A little extra virgin olive oil, especially from a small company that takes special care in pressing their oils, can be helpful for your liver. People who do liver flushes use this oil after a period of fat avoidance to stimulate the gallbladder to contract and flush out gallstones. I no longer recommend the olive oil challenge after fat avoidance type of liver flush because of the possibility of stressing your system beyond repair.

A colleague decided to do a liver flush on general cleansing principles, even though she had no overt signs of liver stress. Doing that flush, however, started a cascade of events that has caused her to become disabled and to give up her practice. If you decide to go ahead with the olive oil challenge after fat avoidance type of flush, I would highly recommend first doing a Functional Liver Detoxification Profile with Great Smokies Diagnostic Laboratory to analyze the functional capacity of your liver. If your liver is having a challenge with detoxifying the toxins you are exposed to, you would benefit from a more gentle cleanse and the support of a health care practitioner. (See Appendix 1 for more information.)

Drinking lemon squeezed into water first thing in the morning is a good tonic for your liver. You may also add fresh-squeezed lemon to your water throughout the day for a refreshing alkalizing drink. Stress and the Standard American Diet (SAD) make your body acidic. An alkalizing cordial and some of the relaxation techniques recommended in Chapter 14 help neutralize acid build up which leads to dysfunction and disease in your body.

In the case of breaking up gallstones, however, mallic acid from apples is helpful. This acid softens the sludge in your gallbladder so that it flows more easily into your small intestine, then out of your body through elimination. Mallic acid is available in all apple products such as applesauce, unfiltered apple juice, and baked, poached, or raw apples. It is not present in filtered apple juices.

A combination of equal parts of fennel, anise, and fenugreek seed tea is cleansing to the liver and soothing to your digestive tract. The time you take to brew the tea and drink it can also be a time of quiet reflection and relaxation which will benefit your health.

Nutritional Products for Liver Cleansing

For an added cleansing bonus, you may opt to add nutritional products to your liver cleanse program. There is plenty of research, as was discussed in Chapter 9, to show the efficacy of milk thistle, also called Silymarin, in liver support. It is available in tincture, tablet, and capsule forms in health food stores. Look for a standardized extract, which will ensure the potency of the product that you are buying. The best extracts contain eighty percent Silymarin extract and are gathered wild. Milk thistle is plentiful in South America and, surprisingly, on my California hillside. (For suppliers of these products check Appendix 1.) Some say that taking herbs continuously diminishes their effect. My recommendation is to use the supplement for a period of no more than two months straight. If you have serious deterioration of your liver and need to take milk thistle for a prolonged amount of time, you may try taking weekends off, with the consent of your health care practitioner, to ensure its effectiveness.

A combination vitamin/mineral/amino acid product called "Detoxification Factors" is helpful in supporting liver detoxification. I have not found it to be as effective as engaging in a thorough cleanse (a modified elimination diet devoid of the usual allergens and with therapeutic food powders), but it is an acceptable compromise for those who cannot or do not wish to engage in a more intensive program. Detoxification Factors (Tyler Encapsulations) include the nutrients needed to support both phases of liver detoxification. It is available through health care practitioners' offices.

"Phosfood," a liquid phosphoric acid compound made by Standard Process and available through doctors' offices, helps liquefy the cholesterol-rich sludge that can get trapped in your gallbladder as a result of bad diet and impaired gastrointestinal function. Please use this product only under the supervision of a licensed health care professional.

Because different products have different potencies and concentrations, it is impossible for me to recommend a dosage for the above-mentioned products. If you are unsure how to proceed after reading the label directions, ask a knowledgeable clerk or work with the aid a licensed health care professional. The advice I give you is not intended to substitute for medical attention, but intended to be informational only.

Liver Detoxification with Ultra Clear or Ultra Clear Plus

Because some people have sensitivity reactions to herbal products, they are unable to use herbal formulations for cleansing. They would do better with a therapeutic food program using Ultra Clear products. For more information about Ultra Clear products, see Chapter 10: "Therapeutic Food Powders for Cleansing."

CLEANSING THE LYMPH SYSTEM

In the early 1900s, an osteopath named Dr. Chapman found that by rubbing certain spots on his patients' bodies, he could relieve their pain and improve the health of their organs. These spots became known as Chapmans' or Neurolymphatic Reflexes. (For more information, see Appendix 1.)

Exercising the Lymph System

One of the best exercises for stimulating lymphatic flow is bouncing on a mini-trampoline jogger. The heel of your foot goes lower than the ball of your foot while you are bouncing on the mini-trampoline. Because of this pulling action, it is perhaps the most effective type of exercise for your lymph system and it also stimulates circulation. Your lymph does not have a pump like your blood vessels have with your heart. The only direct way to get the lymph system to increase its flow, other than by skin brushing (see Chapter 15) and massage, is to exercise. When the big muscles of your body contract with exercise, it squeezes your lymph vessels and improves fluid flow.

Of course any form of exercise or movement beyond sitting on the couch and surfing channels with the remote is helpful for encouraging lymph circulation. When you move, muscles in your body contract and release, squeezing the blood and lymph vessels inside.

CHAPTER 12

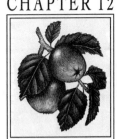

MAINTAINING HEALTHIER BOWELS

BOWEL MOVEMENT PROGRESS CHART

Following is a chart that will help you monitor the results of
your own cleansing program. I suggest you begin your diary
a few days before the beginning of your cleansing program.
This will help you see the dramatic difference that cleansing
makes in your daily elimination. If you wish to continue
your diary beyond four weeks, just make a photocopy of the
page. This is your personal diary, and it will be a valuable
motivational tool to keep you inspired to cleanse. Things to
watch for and to note on your chart are:

- unusual colors of stool
- amount and bulkiness of stool
- sticky vs. dry stool
- firm vs. loose stool
- floating vs. non-floating stool
- mucus strands or pockets
- other items expelled with stool

DAY	1st Bowel Movement	2nd Bowel Movement	3rd Bowel Movement	4th Bowel Movement	5th Bowel Movement
SUNDAY	TIME: DESCRIPTION:	TIME: DESCRIPTION:	TIME: DESCRIPTION:	TIME: DESCRIPTION:	TIME: DESCRIPTION:
MONDAY	TIME: DESCRIPTION:	TIME: DESCRIPTION:	TIME: DESCRIPTION:	TIME: DESCRIPTION:	TIME: DESCRIPTION:
TUESDAY	TIME: DESCRIPTION:	TIME: DESCRIPTION:	TIME: DESCRIPTION:	TIME: DESCRIPTION:	TIME: DESCRIPTION:
WEDNESDAY	TIME: DESCRIPTION:	TIME: DESCRIPTION:	TIME: DESCRIPTION:	TIME: DESCRIPTION:	TIME: DESCRIPTION:
THURSDAY	TIME: DESCRIPTION:	TIME: DESCRIPTION:	TIME: DESCRIPTION:	TIME: DESCRIPTION:	TIME: DESCRIPTION:
FRIDAY	TIME: DESCRIPTION:	TIME: DESCRIPTION:	TIME: DESCRIPTION:	TIME: DESCRIPTION:	TIME: DESCRIPTION:
SATURDAY	TIME: DESCRIPTION:	TIME: DESCRIPTION:	TIME: DESCRIPTION:	TIME: DESCRIPTION:	TIME: DESCRIPTION:

Figure 12.1   **Weekly Bowel Movement Record**

Constipation and Laxatives

Forty million Americans currently use laxatives, and eight million use them at least once a week. Most of these are stimulant laxatives that work by irritating the walls of the intestinal tract, causing increased movement of the colon walls as the body attempts to expel the laxative. With continued use, this results in poor muscle tone, faulty peristalsis, and a further dependence on laxatives. In fact, many people who overuse laxatives reach the point where they are incapable of having a bowel movement without resorting to the use of laxatives, enemas, or colonics. Laxative overuse can also lead to depletion of potassium and other nutrients in the body, as well as to kidney damage in extreme cases.

When constipation does occur, I recommend use of a high-fiber supplement to provide bulk and moisture for smooth elimination rather than turning to stimulant laxatives (see Chapters 3 and 7 for more information on dietary fiber). Wheat bran has become popular for achieving regularity, but with repeated use it tends to be harsh and even irritating to the intestinal tact. Also the phytate in wheat bran forms strong bonds with iron and other minerals, thereby reducing their absorption into the body. Psyllium husks are one of the best types of fiber available. They act gently as they form soft, bulky stools, and they are more efficient at removing waste and toxins from the digestive system than other forms of fiber. In rare cases, it may become necessary to consult with an M.D. if working with these recommendations and an alternative health care practitioner has not yielded the results you need.

Sometimes peristalsis just won't work either; it does not occur or is ineffective. If this is the case, drug intervention may be necessary. Waning hormones may also be responsible for a sluggish bowel, as I have mentioned earlier. To support the hormone estrogen's activity, you can add soy products to your diet on a daily basis in the form of tofu, soy milk, soy burgers (one of my staples while finishing the manuscript for this book), soy nuts, tempeh, miso, and so on. Insufficient thyroid hormone activity may also be responsible for a sluggish intestinal tract. Many natural therapies are now available that can increase the secretion of your own hormones and protect the ones that are being produced. A Health Coach, chiropractor, acupuncturist, naturopath, or certified clinical nutritionist may be able to help you in this area. A few medical doctors are also learning about these less invasive and less harmful ways to support hormone balance, although some will freely admit that their patients know more in this area than they do.

It is in your best interest to prevent problems from occurring by maintaining a high-fiber diet and healthy intestinal flora, and by performing a thorough internal cleansing periodically to remove old encrusted waste and improve the health of your elimination system and your entire body. (See Chapter 7 for more on high-fiber diet and healthy intestinal flora.)

A NOTE ON COLONICS

A colonic is an enema done with water under pressure, which allows the water to penetrate farther into the large intestine. The colonic is administered by a technician who regulates the water pressure. During an internal cleansing program, an occasional enema or a series of colonics can be helpful in removing impacted waste from the colon, relieving constipation, and assisting the cleansing process. Colonic therapists have found that colonics by themselves are not completely effective in removing the long-term putrefactive matter that has adhered to the intestinal walls for years. However, in conjunction with an herbal cleansing, colonics shorten the time required to remove loosened, impacted matter from the colon wall. Many colonic therapists recommend an herbal cleansing to their patients and are amazed at the amount and content of toxic material released by combining internal cleansing with colonics.

It is easy to disrupt the valuable population of bifidobacteria (bifs) and lactobacteria and to introduce a foreign species that may even lead to death when doing colonics, so precautions must be taken. Make sure the colon therapist uses tubes that are new—and reserved only for you if you return for repeat colonics. Always use properly filtered or distilled water rather than spring or chlorinated water. Spring water may contain unknown microorganisms that could damage your health. When you take water in through your mouth, your digestive juices have the chance to kill off any potential pathogens. But with a colonic, the water is going up the back end of your digestive tract, so you don't have that digestive advantage. And chlorinated water kills off the good bacteria in your intestines. After all, isn't that the job of chlorine in our drinking water—to kill microorganisms? If your therapist does not follow your internal washing with an "implant" of beneficial bacteria, follow the enema or colonic with some of the probiotic supplements mentioned in Chapter 14. These may be taken orally.

"GOOD" BACTERIA

Lactobacilli and *bifidobacteria* (bifs) are our friends. They play a significant role in controlling the pH of the large intestine through the liberation of lactic acid and acetic acid, which in turn restrict the growth of potential pathogens in your gut. Their supportive properties may include production of organic acids that inhibit the growth of certain undesirable bacteria, promotion of normal gastrointestinal function, and promotion of a healthy intestinal wall, to name a few. Bifs are believed to have cancer-protective and cholesterol-lowering properties, as well as the ability to synthesize B-vitamins and vitamin K. All beneficial bacteria are susceptible to eradication, especially through the use of any antibiotics. Sugar in your diet in the form of sweeteners and alcohol supports the overgrowth of yeast such as candida, which damages your intestinal wall and leads to allergies and toxicity. These yeasts can mimic your own cells so that your immune system begins to attack your thyroid gland, heart, or other vital body parts. This simple habit of eating too much sugar or having too many alcoholic drinks can lead to autoimmune disease.

PART IV:
STAY CLEAN AND ENJOY VIBRANT GOOD HEALTH

CHAPTER 13

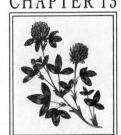

Diet and Recipes That Complement Cleansing

"The goal in life is to die young—as late as possible." — *Ashley Montague, Ph.D.*

What to Eat?

Because we all have different food preferences, I do not recommend one nutritional plan for everyone. Rather, I have compiled a list of recommendations that you may incorporate into your daily diet. These suggestions will help you develop a meal plan as a basis for keeping your intestinal tract clean. (If you wish, you may follow the suggested menus on pages 215–218.)

1. Drink plenty of plain, pure water every day. If you do not yet have a source of purified water, it is better, in most circumstances, to drink tap water than not to drink water at all. (See "Dirty Water," page 90.)

2. Eat plenty of fresh vegetables. They are easy to digest and they provide essential nutrients and

fiber. Vegetable juices are excellent for cleansing your body. Choosing organically grown vegetables is, of course, your best course of action.

3. Eat plenty of fresh fruit. Fruit is high in vitamins and easy to digest, and it helps cleanse your body. Keep intake of fruit to a minimum if you are hypoglycemic or carbohydrate intolerant (see "Determining Your Sensitivity to Insulinogenic Foods and Eating Habits," Chapter 8) — especially sweet fruit such as bananas, sweet melon, dates, and grapes. Again, organically grown fruit is your best choice.

4. Eat whole grains if you tolerate them. People with AB blood types have the least trouble. Whole grains (as opposed to refined grains) are high in dietary fiber and contain an acceptable balance of proteins, carbohydrates, vitamins, minerals, and natural oils. Try adding some grains that are new to North Americans to your diet. Quinoa and amaranth are ancient grains from South America. They are higher in protein than our standard wheat, corn, and rice, and because you were probably not exposed to them in your tender youth, they are unlikely to cause sensitivities or allergies in your system. In the following pages, I have included recipes that incorporate both of these nourishing grains.

5. Eat more sprouted grains, beans, and seeds. They are excellent sources of enzymes, protein, and fiber. They are packed with vitamins and minerals as an added bonus. Because they are "alive" your body has an easier time digesting and assimilating sprouted foods. If you have a weak digestive

system, you may not be able to tolerate raw food. If that is the case, steam your sprouts, vegetables, and fruits to a tenderness suitable to the current health of your digestive tract.

6. Eat plenty of beans and soy products. They are high in protein and fiber, and are an excellent complement to grains. To reduce the gas-forming properties of beans, you can use a product called Bean-O. It contains the enzyme *raphinose*, which breaks down the indigestible fiber portion of beans that causes gas. The macrobiotic community also claims that cooking a couple of sheets of kombu seaweed at the bottom of your pot of beans helps to eliminate gas. Be sure to soak the dry beans, then throw out the soaking water and rinse the beans to assist this process. Since I don't eat many dairy products, and I rarely have an egg, I have invented some whipped cream substitutes and pudding recipes using tofu (which is made from soybeans) to satisfy those desires for creamy, sweet food. (See recipes on pages 210–211.)

7. Eat raw, organically grown nuts and seeds. They are high in protein, oils, and valuable minerals. They are best eaten in moderation—no more than a handful at any one time—because they are so concentrated. Whole nuts that still contain their germ lend themselves to sprouting. Sunflower seeds with the shells on can be grown like a grass; they make a delicious, nutty sprout treat (often available in supermarkets or health food stores). Raw almonds, hazelnuts, and sunflower seeds without the shell are more digestible if soaked

overnight in pure water. Organically grown nuts are much healthier than nuts grown with pesticides, and they should be stored in your freezer or refrigerator in a tightly sealed container to protect their abundant oils from becoming rancid. If you have herpes, you may want to strictly limit your intake of nuts and seeds. (Note: nuts, seeds, and grains, especially corn, are high in *arginine,* which feeds the herpes virus. You can counteract the arginine by taking lysine tablets or capsules and/or eating yogurt.)

8. Eat plenty of cultured or fermented dairy products such as yogurt, kefir, and buttermilk if you tolerate them. If you are unsure, buy a small container as a trial. They are easier to digest than milk, and they usually contain lactobacteria that are beneficial to your intestinal tract. Remember to get organic or nonfat versions that say "live cultures" on the label for your best health.

9. Eat fish. They are a good source of protein and essential fatty acids. Since our planet is increasingly polluted, there are concerns (especially for pregnant women) about the toxins that are concentrated in fish. We discussed at length the dangers of eating any fish from the Great Lakes. However, ocean fish generally have a high concentration of selenium which binds the toxins and makes them harmless to your body when you eat them. You can also buy farm-raised fish, which may be a cleaner product. Call your fish market and ask what the farm-raised fish are fed. If they are fed fish pellets made from mackerel, cod,

herring, or other fish, then your fish should be fine. If they are fed grains or chicken parts, don't buy them. If you do regular cleansing, eat a diet high in EFAs, fruit, and vegetables, drink pure water, and think good thoughts, the benefits of eating fish two to four times per week will probably outweigh the dangers you may encounter. Choose the high-EFA fish that I recommended in Chapter 3.

10. Take a fiber supplement, a probiotic formula, and omega-3 EFAs such as flax oil or docosahexaenoic acid (DHA), or eicosapentaenoic acid (EPA) daily for a well-balanced nutritional program. It is unlikely that modern food will give you all of the nutrition you need for optimum health even if you are mindful of your diet. The benefits of these supplements have been discussed in detail in Chapters 3, 7, and 9.

PHYTONUTRIENTS

Phyto comes from a Greek word meaning "plant." *Phytonutrients* are plant-derived substances that are highly active in the body. Over 20,000 such nutrients in plants have been identified; they not only give plants their bright colors, but also protect the plants and those of us who eat them from environmental stressors. A diet rich in fresh fruits, vegetables, nuts, seeds, grains, and legumes contains hundreds of special compounds that promote good health and are associated with a lowered risk of heart disease, diabetes, high blood pressure, obesity, and cancer. Phytonutrients help reduce our risk of developing these conditions and diseases through antioxidant activity, hormone regulation, suppression of inflammatory pathways, and support of detoxification pathways that flush out carcinogens.

In a 1992 article titled "The Role of Dietary Phytosterols in Colon Carcinogenesis" that appeared in *Nutrition and Cancer,* researchers headed by A.V. Rao stated, "For most cancer sites, persons with low fruit and vegetable intake (at least the lower one-fourth of the population) experience about twice the risk of cancer compared with those with high intake, even after control for potentially confounding factors." A study being undertaken by Britain's Imperial Cancer Research Fund and the Medical Research Council finds, after seventeen years, that people who eat fresh fruit daily are twenty-four percent less likely to die from a heart attack; strokes decrease by thirty-two percent, and twenty-one percent are less likely to die in any given year.

In addition to their individual healing properties, most phytonutrients are antioxidants that trap pollution particles known as *free radicals.* They have also been shown to stop cancer-causing enzymes from performing their dastardly work.

HEALING FOODS FROM NATURE'S BOUNTY

What colors show up on your table? Here are some examples of foods' healing properties:

Red grapes, blackberries, blueberries, and cherries get their royal colors from *anthocyanins,* powerful antioxidants that dilate blood vessels, aid vision, and may help prevent heart disease and stroke.

Blackberries, blueberries, raspberries, and strawberries possess a trio of nutrients—phenolic acids, catechins, and flavonoids—that trap free radicals, stop harmful enzymes, and normalize hormones. Flavonoids also protect your eyes and your heart.

Kiwi fruit has three hundred times as much vitamin C as a comparable weight of oranges, and it is loaded with potassium and the good enzymes bromelain and *papain*, which help injured tissue to heal. Kiwis are also effective at removing excess sodium from the body, which is helpful for people with sodium-dependent high blood pressure.

Mint contains powerful phytonutrients (plant nutrients) called monoterpenes, antioxidants that stimulate protective enzyme production. It is easy to grow mint in a pot or in your yard for a fresh supply whenever you want it. Citrus peel and caraway seeds are other monoterpene food sources.

Peaches and melons grace us with beta-carotene, which is also present in other yellow and orange fruits and vegetables, as well as in leafy greens. Researchers think that beta-carotene is a marker for a wide range of other phytonutrients. There are six hundred known carotenoid antioxidants. Honeydew melons have blood-thinning properties to protect your cardiovascular system.

Citrus fruits feed you folic acid in addition to their well-known vitamin C content. They also contain liminoids and terpenes, which stimulate protective enzymes, including ones that block carcinogenic activities in your body. Later in this chapter, look for some delicious recipes high in these colorful and nutrition-packed foods.

Broccoli, cauliflower, cabbage, and brussels sprouts are cruciferous vegetables that contain the phytonutrients indole and sulforaphane. Indoles may support healthy estrogen metabolism in your body, thereby helping to protect you against breast and ovarian cancers. Sulforaphanes support the removal of toxins and carcinogens, protecting your DNA from damage.

Soybeans contain phytoestrogens that may help to normalize your body's hormonal balance. In this way, they may protect against hormone-related cancers such as breast and prostate cancer. In countries where a lot of soybean foods are consumed, there is a low incidence of hormone-related cancers.

Garlic, onions, leeks, and chives contain allyl sulfides that support cardiovascular health and optimal cholesterol levels. Some studies link these foods to a lower incidence of stomach and colon cancer as well.

Green tea is rich in polyphenols—bioflavonoids with powerful antioxidant properties. It is a favorite beverage of the Japanese, who have a low incidence of gastric cancers.

Tomatoes, red grapefruit, watermelon, and apricots are full of lycopenes—antioxidants with twice the activity of beta-carotene. A study reported in the *International Journal of Cancer* showed that the group of people who ate the most tomatoes had half the risk of digestive tract cancers (mouth, throat, esophagus, stomach, colon, and rectal cancers) as that of the group who ate the least. Another study found that men who ate at least ten servings of tomato-based foods per week reduced their risk of developing prostate cancer by forty-five percent.

Carrots, corn, pumpkin, and squash are high in beta-carotene. Diets rich in this nutrient have been linked to a reduced risk of heart disease and cancer. Beta-carotene promotes the production of vitamin A, which supports your immune system.

Spinach, collard greens, kale, and parsley are rich in another class of carotenoids: lutein and zeaxanthin. These are pigments found in the macula of your eyes. The macula is in the central part of the retina and contains the greatest concentration of nerve cells so that you can see. Macular degeneration is a major cause of blindness in the elderly. If you have this condition, you lose the central part of your vision and can only see in the periphery or outside edges of your field of vision. An article published in the *Journal of the American Medical Association* showed a relationship between macular degeneration and diets low in lutein and zeaxanthin.

Herbs have a variety of phytonutrients that have been used to restore health throughout the ages. Some more widely recognized herbs are ginger, milk thistle, turmeric, echinacea, dong quai, and ginkgo. These herbs have traditionally been used as anti-spasmodics or to support the liver and the digestive and immune systems. Some herbs are known for their use as adaptogens—nutrients that help us adapt to the physical and mental stressors of a modern lifestyle.

Astragalus root, aloe vera, and many Chinese mushrooms contain polysaccharides, which support immune-system function.

Horseradish, mustard, cabbage, turnips, and cashew nuts contain isothiocyanates, which support detoxification and removal of carcinogens.

Lentils and beans are rich in saponins, which help reduce the growth of cancer cells.

Spirulina, chlorella, and dunaliella are "superfoods" in a class called microalgae. They contain a wide range of the amino acids, carbohydrates, EFAs, vitamins, and minerals we need to support life. They are the richest known source of vegetarian B_{12}. Microalgae are the lowest food on the food chain, making life out of only sunlight, water, and the minerals floating in the aquatic environment in which they grow. The addition of microalgae to my diet was one of the most significant steps I have ever taken toward improving my health.

Flower pollen is another superfood that provides protein, carbohydrates, EFAs, enzymes, coenzymes, vitamins, and minerals. It also contains flavonoids, polyphenols, carotenoids, and other phytonutrients. Many people who eat this superfood report improved energy levels.

ALOE VERA

The aloe vera plant is a succulent and a member of the lily family. Aloe vera leaves are filled with a healthful inner gel that contains many valuable nutrients, including vitamins, minerals, enzymes, lipids (fats), amino acids, and healing *mucopolysaccharides*. Aloe vera has been known for centuries as an overall curative and an almost "miracle working" plant. Dioscorides, a medical practitioner in the first century A.D., made a detailed report on aloe for treating wounds, insomnia, stomach disorders, general pain, constipation, and many other disorders. But Western civilization lost the knowledge of aloe as a healing substance until recently.

During the last fifty years, much research on aloe vera has been undertaken to determine why it was so valued throughout history. The studies reveal that aloe vera is very effective in supporting the process of healing from many ailments, including burns, gum disease, and hemorrhoids. One of the greatest benefits of aloe vera juice is the soothing and cleansing effect it has on the whole digestive system. It relieves inflammation of the stomach, especially in the case of ulcers. Research has also shown that aloe inhibits the growth of both staphylococcus and coliform bacteria—the "bad guys"—and promotes the growth of the good lactobacteria that are essential for good digestion.

Aloe vera is particularly beneficial when following an internal cleansing program. At the beginning and for several weeks after ending a program, take two to four ounces of aloe vera juice per day. This juice will help reduce gas and digestive-system irritation, and create an ideal environment for a healthy intestinal tract. I recommend Aloe Falls Aloe Juice, which comes in three varieties: 100% Whole Leaf, Hawaiian Ginger, and Aloe Juice Formula. There are many aloe juices on the market. What distinguishes Aloe Falls is that it is the only aloe vera without preservatives, *and* it is certified active. Yerba Prima makes and distributes Aloe Falls aloe juices.

Yerba Prima had independent laboratory analysis done on Aloe Falls juice at the University of Rhode Island. Cell culture testing was done to verify that the finished products helped promote healthy cell growth. When measuring the activity of aloe, that is the principal question to consider since the juice is used to cleanse and heal your intestinal lining. All three varieties passed the test and were stronger than any other aloe juice on the market. Use discretion when choosing an aloe vera juice; some have harmful bacteria in them, and one had no measurable aloe vera in the product at all. You will find that Aloe Falls is more tasty then other brands as well.

The 100% Whole Leaf Aloe Juice is, of course, the strongest because it has the highest concentration of polysaccharides. Without preservatives, it contains only a little vitamin C to ensure freshness. It is the juice of choice for immune-system problems or for direct application to the skin, and it has the strongest healing effects. If you are suffering with ulcers, this would be the juice to include in your cleansing program. Other whole-leaf aloes may not discard the yellow portion, called *aloin*, that lies between the rind and the gel. Aloin has strong laxative properties and interferes with the healing properties of the rest of the plant.

Hawaiian Ginger Aloe Juice contains fifty percent aloe vera gel and fifty percent Hawaiian ginger and white grape juice. It has a warming effect, supports digestive function, and is an anti-inflammatory, supporting the anti-inflammatory effects of aloe. This would be the beverage of choice if you have a sluggish digestive system as indicated by a puffy tongue with scalloped edges. You might pause for a moment right now and go check this out in a mirror.

Aloe Juice Formula is fifty percent aloe vera gel and fifty percent extracts from teas of peppermint, chamomile, and parsley tea extracts. It is more cooling than the ginger formula, and may be helpful for those with Irritable Bowel Syndrome (IBS). Enteric-coated peppermint (peppermint coated with a substance to delay release until it hits the small intestines) has been shown to relieve symptoms of IBS. Peppermint works both in the stomach and in the intestines. Chamomile has been used for centuries as a calming herb, and parsley is mildly diuretic, helping expel excess water. As I mentioned earlier, parsley and all leafy green vegetables are high in magnesium—a relaxer for your entire system.

Look for recipes including these healthful beverages later in this chapter.

BENTONITE

Bentonite is a natural clay mineral that exists as discrete deposits in most continents of the world. It was created primarily in volcanic eruptions millions of years ago, when the volcanic ash settled in shallow seas and eventually became bentonite clay. Some of the largest deposits are found in the Great Plains area of the United States.

There are two major types of bentonite, identified by the major exchangeable ion present in the clay. Those higher in sodium, as opposed to calcium, have greater beneficial activity. In its purified form, bentonite is free of all contamination. It passes through your body undigested. This clay is composed of numerous microscopic platelets, each with negative charges on the flat surfaces and positive charges on the edges. When properly hydrated, the water molecules cause these platelets to separate into a porous structure containing both negative and positive charges. This swelling allows bentonite to absorb substances in the space between the platelets. The ionic charges give bentonite the ability to bind toxins and hold them until they are eliminated. The structure of Great Plains bentonite creates an enormous surface—over nine hundred square yards per tablespoon—that traps and binds pesticides and other potentially harmful substances so that they do not remain in your body.

Montmorillonite, the principal constituent of bentonite, is used in many industries, including water treatment, cosmetics, pharmaceuticals, and dietary supplements. Tested against other clays, including kaolin, which can be found in Kaopectate, low concentrations of montmorillonite were more effective than high concentrations of other clays in suppressing the activity of a highly infectious fungus called *histoplasma capsulatum* that is present in soil and can cause lung diseases and other complications when inhaled.

I am happy to announce that bentonite has been found effective in neutralizing pesticides. It is comforting to know that there is a natural antidote to these dangerous synthetic poisons. Bentonite was shown to be an effective part of treatment for Paraquat (a pesticide) toxicity, and there was a reduction in the toxicity of Roundup (an herbicide) when bentonite was used. In the mid-1970s, the Committee of Scientists of the Agricultural Research Service, USDA (U.S. Department of Agriculture), listed 169 agricultural pesticides used in the United States. Nearly two thirds were shown to be potentially absorbed onto bentonite, neutralizing their toxicity to humans. Aflatoxins—extremely carcinogenic molds found on grains and nuts, especially peanuts—adsorbed better to bentonite clays high in sodium than to those high in calcium.

Bentonite has also been evaluated for its ability to relieve diarrhea. In the 1960s, a liquid solution of bentonite was tested in thirty-five cases of diarrhea caused by virus infection, food allergy, spastic colon, mucous colitis, or food poisoning. The diarrhea cleared up in thirty-four out of the thirty-five cases in an average of four days by taking two tablespoons three times per day. In animal studies in the 1980s, bentonite blocked intestinal absorption of a toxic substance introduced into the food of rats. This toxin is known to cause vomiting, refusal to eat, and gastrointestinal lesions in livestock, poultry, and humans. In another study published in *Gastroenterology*, bentonite was shown to bind to toxins in the blood from E. coli and other sources. The study stated: "The most effective material in the prevention of endotoxemia proved to be bentonite. . . ."

In considering which brand of bentonite to choose to augment your cleansing needs, please consider these factors: ion ratios, activity, and purity. Choose a product that has a higher ratio of sodium to calcium ions. Maximum swelling and binding activity are achieved when the sodium ions comprise sixty-five to seventy-five percent of the total exchangeable ions. Use only the highest grade, which is purified USP/NF (United States Pharmacopoeia/National Formulary). My bentonite of choice is Great Plains Bentonite. It meets or exceeds all of the above criteria. Their purification process goes through four stages. First, water washing removes any nonclay material, and then removes the less effective nonswelling fraction of the clay. Finally, the material is dried, milled, sorted, and then tested extensively to ensure that it exceeds the stringent USP/NF purity standards for microbial limits, absence of pathogens, absence of adulteration, and product consistency. Every batch of Great Plains Bentonite is tested for purity and consistency. I have used other forms of bentonite in the past, and I was impressed by the whiteness of the Great Plains product. Does that mean that the product I used before contained impurities? Probably so. The use of advanced processing methods results in a Great Plains Bentonite surface of over 960 square yards per serving. That is over twelve football fields of surface area per quart bottle!

THE IMPORTANCE OF WATER — *PLENTY* OF WATER

I have discussed the value of pure water extensively in Chapters 3 and 6. If you are not drinking enough water during a cleanse, you will endanger the health of your tissues as concentrated toxins are being eliminated from your cells. Furthermore, dehydration can have deleterious effects on your body, eventually leading to death. Probably few of us are close to that stage of water loss, but if you are experiencing heartburn, rheumatoid pain, back pain, heart or angina pain, headaches, or leg pain from walking, you may be suffering from chronic dehydration.

Joint movement is facilitated by water. The cartilage lining in your joints needs fluid to create a cushion between your bones. Without sufficient water, an inflammatory process can ensue to compensate for the lack of water. It may appear that there is an infection or arthritis in your joints, when in reality there is only dehydration.

In your stomach and duodenum—the first portion of your small intestines—a mucus barrier prevents acid penetration and damage to your gastrointestinal lining. A well-hydrated mucus barrier will retain bicarbonate and neutralize acid as it tries to pass through the mucus. Hydration will provide a much better acid barrier to the mucosa than any medication on the market.

If your double-layer cell membranes lack sufficient water, enzyme movement in and out of your cells will be obstructed. Enzymes are necessary to activate cell functions.

Even hypertension or high blood pressure can be helped by optimal water consumption. When you have inadequate volume in your blood stream, the vessels selectively decrease in diameter. The vascular system adapts to volume loss by selectively closing the blood vessel lumen. One major cause of blood volume loss is insufficient body water. In chronic dehydration, water is lost from inside of some cells, from water volume held outside the cells, and from water held in the blood vessels. The compensatory closing of the lumen to compensate for water loss causes the rise in tension recognized as hypertension.

Drink Half Your Weight in Ounces of Water Every Day

If you weigh 160 pounds, you would benefit by drinking eighty ounces of water each day. Or if you weigh two hundred pounds, then drink one hundred ounces of water. The tallest water bottles available at grocery stores contain approximately fifty-two ounces of water. If you weigh 104 pounds, that would be the amount of water that would benefit you most. You can get also get water in fruit juices, teas, sparkling water, and soda, but each of them has a distinct disadvantage. When you drink juice, you are requiring the digestive machinery and the pancreas to fire up and work. Drinking pure water allows your body to flush out toxins without having to mobilize your digestive system.

Tea of the caffeinated kind is actually a diuretic. By drinking caffeinated teas, coffee, colas, and chocolate drinks you are depleting the supply of water available in your body to dilute toxins and "moisturize" your system. Herbal teas often have therapeutic effects that also make your body work instead of giving it a well-deserved rest. Some herbal teas, such as parsley tea, are also diuretic in action.

Sparkling water may have a high level of phosphorus, which can interfere with calcium absorption in your body and contribute to the development of osteoporosis—something we all want to avoid.

Soda is in a class by itself. Read the ingredients; they might not be what you want to put in your body. Many sodas are "rich" with toxic synthetic chemicals and caffeine.

One can of soda usually contains *six tablespoons* of sugar. In addition, soda may also be high in phosphorus.

Some people have difficulty drinking water. Here are some suggestions that may help:

1. Drink from a small juice glass in small sips throughout the day.
2. Put fresh-squeezed lemon in your water. It then becomes an alkalinizing treat to help neutralize the acid of many diseases, disorders, or conditions. This drink will help normalize your pH, enhancing all of the metabolic processes that your body performs every second of your life. Patients who formerly drank a lot of soda told me that they enjoyed this unsweetened lemonade so much that they didn't feel deprived from giving up their soda. If you use Meyer lemons, which are sweeter than normal lemons, you automatically add to the deliciousness of this tasty beverage and you gain the benefit of the naturally occurring vitamin C with your lemon-charged water.
3. Put a slice of cucumber in your water. I was first introduced to this refreshing drink in a Mexican restaurant. It is also slightly alkalizing.
4. Mix a fruit juice that you like with an equal amount of water. That way you cause less of a digestive reaction, enjoy a taste sensation that you like, and benefit from increased water consumption. You may find that, as you become accustomed to this new taste, you will be able to increase the amount of water while decreasing the proportion of juice.

5. Soak in a tub of water. Did you ever notice how you have to urinate after swimming or soaking in water? You absorb water through your skin, which is why it is so important to bathe, soak, or shower in high-quality water.

Getting good nutrition can be delicious and fun. Following are a few favorite recipes that help me enjoy nutrient-rich and scrumptious meals. Feel free to improvise. Let your intuition and what is available and appealing at the market be your guides to preparing delicious, nutritious food for you and your loved ones.

ANTIOXIDANT SALADS

You know by now the importance of having a diet rich in antioxidant nutrients to combat the effects of toxicity from whatever the source: the environment, your own digestive system, or your home or workplace. Eating ripe fruit and vegetables in season is one of the best ways to fulfill this need. If ripe produce is not available, you may purchase frozen fruits and vegetables; these foods are often frozen within hours of picking. Some argue that quick-frozen food is fresher than produce purchased at the supermarket, since supermarket food has been kept in storehouses and shipped across the country or the world before it finally reaches your table. The best way to be assured of the quality of the food you eat is to grow your own. Since that plan doesn't fit into many busy lifestyles, a local farmers' market is the next best option.

A word about organically grown versus commercially grown produce: organic is better. Some organically grown foods boast a nutrient density as much as ninety percent higher than commercially grown foods. In order to look pretty and sell quickly, foods require a minimum level of nutrients in the soil in which they grow. This does not ensure that they will have the nutrients necessary to make a human being healthy. Organically grown food usually costs more than commercially grown food, but considering that, on average, it has fifty percent more nutrition than commercial produce, the higher cost is well worth the price. As a bonus, organically grown produce is free of harmful pesticides. Refer to Chapter 5 for a discussion of the dangers of pesticides.

Antioxidant Fruit Salad

Yield: 3 to 6 servings

> 2 oranges *or* 1 grapefruit, peeled and sliced
> 2 kiwis, chopped into bite-size pieces
> 2 bananas, chopped into bite-size pieces
> 2 crisp apples, cored and sliced (peeled optional)
> 1 cup blueberries, fresh or *frozen
> 1 fresh pineapple, chopped into bite-size pieces
> 1 cup halved strawberries, fresh or *frozen
> 1 mango, chopped into bite-size pieces

Place the oranges (or grapefruit) and the kiwi in a bowl. Then mix in the other ingredients. The ascorbic acid from the citrus and kiwi will coat the rest of the fruit and protect it from oxidizing (turning brown).

This delicious salad is high in vitamin C, vitamin A, beta-carotene, fiber, *acanthosides* from the blueberries (good for vision), antifungal substances from the banana, and proteolytic enzymes from the pineapple, which can kill parasites and decrease pain and inflammation, plus whatever other great nutrients we have yet to discover.

Note: If some of the fruit is frozen, mix together first and microwave up to 2 minutes or heat over a double boiler until softened, then mix in with the other fruit.

Antioxidant Vegetable Salad

Yield: 2 to 4 servings

> 1 to 2 grated or thinly sliced carrots
> ½ onion, thinly sliced or diced *or* 1 to 2 green onions, diced
> 1 to 2 stalks celery, thinly sliced
> 1 small cucumber, sliced or cubed
> 1 red or green pepper, sliced or diced
> 1 head broccoli, chopped into florets, raw or slightly steamed

Mix all ingredients together. You can serve this vegetable salad on a bed of raw lettuce or cooked greens.

This salad is high in vitamin A, vitamin C, beta-carotene, flavonoids from the onion, and anticarcinogenic substances from the broccoli, plus whatever else Mother Nature has provided for us that we don't know about yet!

Lemon and Garlic Salad Dressing

Yield: about 1½ cups

> ½ cup flaxseed oil
> ½ cup sesame *or* olive oil
> 1 to 2 cloves garlic, crushed or diced
> Juice of 1 lemon *or* 2 limes
> Splash of your favorite vinegar (optional)
> Salt, tamari, soy sauce, or Bragg's Liquid Aminos
>   (non-fermented), to taste
> Freshly ground pepper, to taste

Whip together or blend all ingredients, and pour over salad. You may add some mustard or nut butter for a different taste or texture. Sunflower and sesame butter (tahini) are two of my favorites. Avoid peanut butter, since its fat suppresses immune-system function.

The essential fatty acids (EFAs) from the oils and seeds are immunity boosting, heart protective, anti-inflammatory, and hormone regulating to enhance your health.

Poppy Seed Dressing

Yield: 6 servings

This recipe and the next two dressings come from Health Coach's Guilt Free Indulgence Cookbook. They are all delicious and, with the addition of flaxseed oil, boost your daily supply of health-enhancing EFAs.

Use this dressing for any salad, pita pocket, potato, or pasta salad. Keep the extra dressing in a dark bottle in the refrigerator for future use.

2 tablespoons honey
2 tablespoons sesame seeds
1 tablespoon poppy seeds
1½ teaspoons chopped white onion
¼ teaspoon wheat-free tamari/soy sauce *or* Worcester-
    shire sauce
¼ teaspoon paprika
¼ cup flaxseed oil
¼ cup sunflower oil
¼ cup cider vinegar (replace with tarragon vinegar or
    lemon juice for variety)

Simply combine all ingredients in a blender or food processor and process until smooth.

Ginger Dressing

Yield: about ¼ cup

This light dressing is great over grains, lettuce, vegetables, coleslaw, or any other salad. You couldn't ask for anything simpler.

3 tablespoons flaxseed oil
1 to 2 tablespoons freshly squeezed lemon juice
1 teaspoon freshly grated ginger
1 clove garlic, minced

Place ingredients in a bowl and whisk together with a fork or blend a larger quantity of all the ingredients in a blender and retain for future use. Store in a dark bottle in the refrigerator.

Lemon-Orange Dressing

Yield: about 2 cups

Extremely easy to make, this is a dressing that can be used for salads, rice, pasta, or any grain dish. With the lemon and orange juice incorporated, it is a dressing filled with sunshine! If you are sensitive to vinegar yet enjoy some zing, then this is perfect for you.

> ¼ cup fresh-squeezed lemon juice
> 3 tablespoons fresh-squeezed orange juice
> ½ cup sunflower oil
> ½ cup flaxseed oil
> 1 tablespoon dill weed *or* 1 teaspoon dried dill
> 1 tablespoon marjoram
> ½ teaspoon fresh ginger *or* 1 teaspoon ground

Just toss all the ingredients into a blender and mix. Place it in a dark bottle and refrigerate.

Quinoa Salad

Yield: 4 to 6 servings

> 1 cup quinoa, uncooked
> 2 cups pure water
> 1 clove garlic, crushed or diced
> ½ cup diced celery
> ½ cup grated carrot
> 1 rounded teaspoon nutritional yeast (optional)

Place the quinoa in a fine-mesh sieve and rinse well with pure water. Pour quinoa in a medium saucepan and add the pure water. Bring to a boil, then immediately turn down the heat to low. Cook covered for 15 minutes or until all of the water is absorbed. If you want a warm salad, immediately mix in the rest of the ingredients. If you prefer a cold salad, let the quinoa salad cool and refrigerate for at least one hour before eating. For a more mellow flavor, cook the garlic with the quinoa. Toss with your favorite dressing. The *Guilt Free Gourmet* Ginger Dressing (page 199) is an excellent choice here.

HEALTHY GRAINS

These grain recipes are high in omega-3 and omega-6 EFAs.

Instant Hot Cereal

Yield: 2 servings

This simple, fast, yet nutritious cereal from The Guilt Free Gourmet *can be altered quite easily to give you a good variety of flavors. Cool mornings are always a great time for hot cereal, provided you are hungry and looking for something to hold you and yours until noon or at least break time. It is also a favorite afternoon snack.*

> 1½ cups pure water, apple cider, *or* other fruit juice
> Handful of raisins *and/or* chopped almonds, if desired
> 1 tablespoon sesame *or* sunflower seeds
> ½ cup ground grains such as amaranth, brown rice, oat groats, oat bran, millet, buckwheat groats, *or* rye (use one or two of these)

Toppings
>   Cinnamon (optional)
>   Flaxseed oil (optional)
>   Fresh fruit, puréed (optional)

Bring the water, cider, or juice to a boil with the raisins, nuts, and seeds, then add the grains, stirring constantly. Simmer for 5 minutes or until desired texture is achieved, and serve. Top it with cinnamon and flaxseed oil or a little fresh fruit purée, such as apple sauce. Mmmmm!

Note: It's best to grind your own grains in a coffee or seed grinder, but you can purchase ground grains from your health food store.

Blueberry Oatmeal

Yield: 3 or 4 servings

If you enjoy hot oatmeal on those cold, blizzard-struck mornings, then this will be a real treat for you. It can also be made with other fruits such as strawberries, raspberries, or bananas. This is another recipe from The Guilt Free Gourmet.

>   2 cups apple cider
>   1 cup pure water
>   1 cup rolled oats
>   3 tablespoons flaxseeds, ground
>   ½ cup rice cereal *or* short-grain rice (ground in your
>   grinder)
>   Handful of blueberries, raisins, *or* other fruit (fresh or
>   frozen)

Bring the apple cider and water to a boil. Stir in the remaining ingredients and let cook on medium heat for 15 minutes or until done.

Note: Try grinding your own grains in a coffee or seed grinder, or purchase freshly ground grains from your health food store.

Fiber Muffins

Yield: about 2 dozen 2-inch muffins

> 2 cups whole wheat flour
> 1 cup Colon Care Formula or Nutri Flax
> ¾ teaspoon unrefined sea salt
> 1¼ teaspoons baking soda
> 2 cups plain yogurt, nonfat organic
> 1 egg, lightly beaten *or* 2 tablespoons ground flaxseed
>   *or* Nutri Flax
> ¾ cup light-flavor honey *or* maple syrup
> 2 tablespoons soft unsalted butter, ghee (clarified
>   butter), *or* coconut oil
> ¼ to ½ cup pure water, if necessary to thin the batter
> 1 cup raisins *or* chopped prunes

Preheat the oven to 425°F.

Lightly oil a muffin tin or line with paper cups.

In a large bowl, combine the dry ingredients. In another large bowl, beat together the yogurt, egg, honey, and butter. Add dry ingredients and fold in with a few quick strokes. (Add the pure water if necessary.) Fold in the raisins. Fill prepared muffin tin two-thirds full.

Bake 15 to 20 minutes or until done.

Quick Chunky Tomato Sauce

Yield: 4 servings

Eating tomatoes helps protect you from free radicals and trap them. For those who eschew grains for health reasons, I recommend adding fiber to canned soups. It is especially good in tomato or vegetable soup. You may also try adding some additional fiber (Colon Care Formula or Nutri Flax) to tomato sauce, especially if you are eating a refined pasta. Add 1 teaspoon for each 1 to 2 servings.

> 2 tablespoons olive oil
> ¼ cup chopped onion
> 1 clove garlic, crushed or minced
> 1 jar (1 pound, 12 ounces) whole Italian-style plum
>   tomatoes with juices
> 1 cup pure water
> 1 tablespoon plus 1 teaspoon Colon Care Formula
>   (CCF) *or* Nutri Flax (NF)
> 1 tablespoon julienned fresh basil *or* 1 teaspoon dried
> 1 tablespoon torn fresh basil leaves, for garnish
> Salt and fresh ground pepper, to taste

Heat olive oil in a medium skillet; stir in onion. Sauté over low heat until tender, about 5 minutes. Stir in garlic, and sauté 1 minute. Add tomatoes and cook over medium heat, stirring and breaking up the tomatoes with the side of a spoon until boiling. Simmer sauce uncovered until slightly thickened, about 15 minutes. Stir in the pure water and the CCF or NF. Cook for 1 to 2 minutes before adding the basil, salt, and pepper. Toss with hot pasta and garnish with remaining basil leaves. Season and serve.

Gazpacho

Yield: 4 servings of 1 cup each

Here's another tomato offering from Health Coach's Guilt Free Indulgence.

There are many varieties of this Spanish national soup, but this recipe is one of the best and certainly the healthiest. Flavored with fresh herbs, gazpacho supplies plenty of vitamin A and potassium, and is a wonderful soup served cold in the traditional way or, if you prefer, heated up. This soup does not require any cooking, and therefore it retains the vitality of its fresh ingredients and can be "whipped up" in a jiffy. Perfect for those thermos lunches and picnics.

¼ white onion, chopped
⅓ cucumber, peeled and seeded
¼ cup green pepper, chopped
1 clove garlic (or more if desired), chopped
1 teaspoon minced fresh coriander *or* ¼ teaspoon dried
5 ripe tomatoes, unpeeled and chopped
1 (6-ounce) can organic *or* natural tomato juice with no additives
1 tablespoon flaxseed oil
1 tablespoon red wine vinegar *or* lemon juice
Pinch of vegetable seasoning
Dash of Tabasco sauce
4 celery stalks with leaves (use celery hearts), chopped
1 tablespoon minced chives
1 tablespoon minced fresh basil *or* parsley
Celery stalks for garnish

Place all the ingredients except celery, chives, and basil in a blender or food processor and purée until desired consistency (smooth or chunky). Mix the purée with the chopped celery, chives, and basil. Chill and serve along with whole celery stalks in cold soup bowls garnished with herbs. Add more Tabasco sauce, garlic, or cayenne for a spicier soup.

Note: If you want to increase your fiber intake for the day, you can add 2 to 4 teaspoons of CCF or NF to this recipe.

Immunity Boosting Soup

Yield: 6 to 10 servings (or freeze half of the pot for later enjoyment)

The potatoes give this soup a lot of body. Try it plain or with either of the herb seasonings offered. Also, try substituting winter squash for potatoes and adding a sweet cashew nut milk (see Variation page 208).

> 1 onion, sliced or diced
> 5 to 10 cloves garlic, coarsely chopped
> Sesame oil *or* water as needed
> 1 bunch kale, collards, mustard greens, *or* Swiss chard, coarsely chopped
> 3 potatoes, well-scrubbed, chopped into 1-inch cubes
> 2 summer squash *or* zucchini, chopped
> 2 celery stalks, chopped
> 4 to 10 shiitake mushrooms, sliced
> 1 to 1½ quarts soup stock

In a large saucepan, sauté the onion and garlic in oil or water. You may add the other vegetables one at a time to the pan to coat them and seal in the nutrients, or you can immediately add the soup stock to the sautéed onions and garlic. My soup stock is usually the water left over from previously steamed vegetables that I keep frozen in yogurt containers until needed. I don't bother to defrost the stock. I run the container upside-down under water until the frozen mass loosens (like a homemade Popsicle). The frozen stock will melt in the cooking pot after being covered with a lid. When the stock starts to simmer you can add the rest of the vegetables.

Or do it the easy way: cut up all of the vegetables or chop them in a food processor, add the soup stock and veggies to the pot, cover, and cook over medium heat until done (about 30 minutes). Less cooking time is needed if you use a food processor to chop your vegetables, since they will be in smaller pieces. If you use this last method of preparation, be sure to watch the pot and stir the ingredients so that the vegetables don't burn while the frozen stock is melting.

Variation: For a different flavor, substitute 1 acorn or butternut squash, skin removed and cubed, for potatoes.

Two Herb Seasonings for Potato Version of Immunity Boosting Soup

Try either of these recipes with the potato version of Immunity Boosting Soup for more potency and flavor.

1 tablespoon fresh rosemary, finely chopped *or*
  1½ teaspoons dried rosemary
Salt and pepper, to taste

OR

½ teaspoon dried sage
1 to 2 bay leaves
Salt and pepper, to taste

For each recipe, simply blend ingredients together and use as a topping for individual bowls of soup.

Seasoning for Winter Squash Version of Immunity Boosting Soup

If you make this soup with winter squash instead of potatoes, try this seasoning recipe.

1 teaspoon cinnamon
¼ teaspoon cumin
¼ teaspoon nutmeg *or* fresh grated, to taste
Salt and pepper, to taste

Blend all ingredients in a bowl and then sprinkle on top of individual bowls of soup.

Variation: To increase the anticarcinogenic effect of this variety, make a milk of 1 cup cashews by softening them in 2 cups pure water for a few hours. If you don't want to wait or don't have the time, then blend cashews with enough water to make into a milky consistency. You can strain the nut meat out if you like. I prefer to leave it in and get all of the protective nutrients that I can from these sweet nuts.

Note: It is best to grind your pepper fresh, as ground pepper that sits around oxidizes and becomes carcinogenic.

Alkaline Broth

This recipe is good nourishment during a cleanse or anytime. For this recipe, simply put all of the best vegetables you can find into a pot.

Potatoes, well-scrubbed and chopped
Zucchini, chopped
Celery, chopped
Beets, chopped
Swiss chard, chopped
Green beans, chopped
Carrots, chopped
Spinach, chopped
Parsley, chopped
Fresh or dried herbs of your choice, to taste

Place ingredients in a large pot, cover with pure water, and simmer. If you want a fresher, chunkier broth, cook only until vegetables are tender, approximately 10 minutes. Put the entire mixture into a blender or food processor and whirl until a purée consistency.

If you favor a broth, cook the vegetables for up to 60 minutes, strain, and toss the vegetables but not the broth. Savor the broth; it's filled with nutrients. This is nice to put in a thermos and sip throughout the day as an antidote to an acid-forming, stressful schedule.

RECIPES FOR HORMONE SUPPORT

In Chapters 2 and 6, I spoke about the importance of hormone health for the elimination of toxins, and about the benefits of internal cleansing. Following are recipes based on soy products that can help your body make the hormones you need to activate your elimination systems.

Better Than Chocolate Pudding

Yield: 4 servings

> 1 package (8 ounces) firm tofu
> ⅛ to ¼ cup carob powder*
> 6 to 8 large pitted dates**
> 1 teaspoon to 1 tablespoon orange zest
> 1 teaspoon vanilla *or anise* flavoring
> Nuts or fresh fruit slices for garnish

Crumble the tofu into a blender or food processor. Add the carob powder. Blend at medium speed. Blend in dates, orange zest, and flavoring. For a smooth consistency, blend the mixture several times. To preserve your appliance motor, turn it off after 30 seconds, scrape the sides of the container to mix the ingredients thoroughly, and blend again. Refrigerate for 30 minutes before serving if you like your pudding chilled. Top with nuts or slices of fresh fruit.

Note: *You may need to rub the carob through a fine sieve if it is lumpy.

**Take as much skin as possible off of the dates if it is easy. If not, soak them in pure warm water in a covered container for 15 minutes before adding the dates to the rest of the ingredients.

Whipped "Cream," Tofu Style

Yield: 4 servings

I like this whipped cream better than dairy-style because it has more body and holds up much better when mixed with the fruit in recipes such as Fruit Parfait. It also has the advantage of nourishing your hormones without adding cholesterol to your heart, arteries, or veins.

> 1 package (8 ounces) firm tofu
> Juice of ½ small lemon
> ¼ to ½ cup sweetener, to taste
> ¼ to 1 teaspoon vanilla, to taste

Blend all the ingredients together following the recommendations for Better Than Chocolate Pudding.

Fruit Parfait

Yield: 4 servings

> *Here's a chance to be creative and add variety to your diet based on the best of the season or what's available in the freezer compartment.*

> 2 cups fresh fruit, cut into bite-size pieces
> 1 cup nuts
> 1 recipe Whipped "Cream," Tofu Style

Layer fresh cut fruit and/or nuts with the Whipped "Cream," Tofu Style.

Variations: Instead of fruit, try 1 cup applesauce. Once I made a strawberry-rhubarb compote by mixing equal parts of fruit and cooking them over low heat for 15 minutes. I added sweetener to taste for the last 5 minutes of cooking, then let the fruit compote cool before layering with the whipped cream.

Note: In the winter, you can use frozen fruit, but be sure it is well thawed before layering with the whipped cream. To thaw the fruit, microwave it for up to 2 minutes or heat over a double boiler until softened.

Drink Recipes for Total Nutritional Support

Fruit Smoothie

Yield: 1 to 2 servings

One of the easiest ways to get the nutrition from fresh fruit, probiotic formulas, and fiber is to add it all to a smoothie. Use a variety of ingredients to whip up a delicious, nutritious treat extraordinaire.

> 1 cup live-culture nonfat yogurt
> ⅔ cup fresh or frozen fruit
> 1 teaspoon Colon Care Formula *or* Nutri Flax
> 1 teaspoon flaxseed oil
> ¼ teaspoon Ultra Flora Plus
> 1 tablespoon Probioplex Intensive Care
> Sweetener, to taste (if desired)

Place all ingredients in a blender and process until smooth.

Note: If you are sensitive to dairy products, you may use nut, soy, rice, or oat milk available in your health food store, or use more fruit and pure water.

Variations: The aloe juice drinks from Aloe Falls would be an excellent addition here as well. Use 2 to 4 ounces per drink.

Another superfood that I add to my concoction is algae.

If you use brewer's yeast, bee pollen, or Metagenics PhytoPro, you can add them to your smoothie.

Instead of yogurt, I most often use one of the Ultra Clear powders designed by Dr. Bland to ensure that I get good nutrition to start my day.

If you're not sure how it would taste to add all of those unusual ingredients to your smoothie, start simple with one or two additives and work your way up to find the perfect brew for you. If you don't have a blender, mix all of the ingredients in a bowl and enjoy. I omit algae and the Ultra Clear products if I eat this recipe in a bowl (because in a milkshake you aren't staring at the green algae, but in a bowl . . .).

Silly Pudding

Yield: 2 servings

I call this pudding silly because it contains psyllium husks and also because it is pretty untraditional.

8 ounces fruit juice
½ cup soaked organic raisins
2 teaspoons Colon Care Formula *or* Nutri Flax
½ cup sliced bananas
Pure water, if needed for consistency

Shake or blend vigorously the juice, raisins, and CCF or NF in a glass jar or blender. Pour into a bowl and top with banana slices. The fiber will absorb all of the water and congeal to the consistency of pudding in a few minutes. If you like, add some of your favorite flavoring such as vanilla or cinnamon.

Mild Laxative Treats

Yield: 8 to 10 balls

> 1 pint mixed, soaked, and mashed dried fruit such as
>   raisins, prunes, dates, figs, or unsulfured apricots
> 1 ounce carob powder
> 1 ounce ground licorice root
> 1 ounce slippery elm powder
> ½ cup Colon Care Formula *or* Nutri Flax
> Sweetener to taste
> 2 ounces shredded coconut (optional)
> Shredded coconut *or* sesame seeds as needed (toasted
>   if desired), for rolling

In a medium bowl, mix together all ingredients except shredded coconut (or sesame seeds) for rolling. To prevent the dough from sticking to your hands, oil your hands. Roll teapoonfuls of dough into little balls, and then roll them in the coconut or sesame seeds.

Refrigerate or freeze before serving to make them firm.

Suggested Menus

Breakfast

If you need to eat a low-carbohydrate diet, I recommend having a shake of Ultra Clear or Ultra Clear Plus for breakfast for an optimally balanced protein-to-carbohydrate ratio. Just put the powder and pure water into a closed container and shake—you are ready to fly! What could be simpler? If you have chosen to add some of the probiotic formulas, try mixing up a Fruit Smoothie (page 212). This nutritious, quick breakfast will get you well nourished and supercharged to start your day.

If you prefer solid food, but have little time, try a banana, apple, pear, or other fresh fruit coated with a tablespoon of sesame, almond, cashew, or sunflower butter. If you are prone to herpes outbreaks, take a 500-milligram tablet of lysine with this quick and delicious meal. Try not to eat peanuts in any form because they may have an inflammatory effect on your body—unless it is for the sheer joy of the taste of peanut sauce on your food, as in Thai food.

Or try eating like the Asians. Have chicken or fish soup with vegetables for breakfast. This is a little unusual for most Americans, but a good option for carbohydrate-intolerant individuals. This breakfast will keep your motor happily humming for many hours.

If you are able to tolerate and enjoy carbohydrates, try the recipes for Instant Hot Cereal (page 201), Blueberry Oatmeal (page 202), or Fiber Muffins (page 203). People who like this option for breakfast, but don't have the desire or facility to grind the grains, can cook up a big pot of grains in the evening when they have more time and store the leftovers in the refrigerator. In the morning, simply heat up some of the grains in a pot or in the microwave oven with some milk (cow, nut, soy, goat, rice, or oat) for a satisfying and tasty meal. You can make this savory dish even better by adding miso or soy sauce and brewer's yeast, or try spicing it up by adding cayenne or garlic. You might also try sweetening it by adding applesauce, fruit, or raisins, but be careful; many people find that eating fruit and grains together causes intestinal gas. Another variation is to add nuts, keeping in mind that the same caution applies to the nut or seed butter breakfast option: if you get herpes, add a lysine supplement.

If you are the kind of person who does best with a light first meal, you might want to try the Antioxidant Fruit Salad (page 196) or just eat a piece of fresh fruit. Alkaline Broth (page 208) is another breakfast option to consider.

To ensure that you start your day with those health-promoting omega-3 essential fatty acids, add a teaspoon to a tablespoon (depending on your body weight and the doses you will be taking later in the day) of fresh flaxseed oil to a shake, soup, or grain mixture. Remember, never cook with fresh flaxseed oil; add the oil to a soup or grain dish after placing it in a bowl to eat.

Lunch

If you want to lose weight, lunch should be your biggest meal of the day. Having most of your calories at this meal gives you ample time to burn off excess calories with your activities of the day. A short walk—even marching in place while returning calls—after lunch sets up your metabolism to burn more effectively for hours when you do finally sit down and get to work.

For a lunch that will power you through your afternoon, try the Antioxidant Vegetable Salad (page 197) with a piece of tofu, fish, or chicken. For a tasty salad dressing, try Lemon and Garlic (page 198), Poppy Seed (page 198), Ginger (page 199), or Lemon-Orange Dressing (page 200).

For a more complex carbohydrate meal, try Quinoa Salad (page 200) with any of the dressings mentioned above to ensure a dose of omega-3 and omega-6 essential fatty acids with your noontime meal.

Quick Chunky Tomato Sauce (page 204) on top of potatoes, cooked grains, or whole grain pasta is a welcome taste treat for lunch. If you are carbohydrate-intolerant, simply serve the sauce on top of tuna, fish, chicken, or beans.

Gazpacho (page 205) or Immunity Boosting Soup (page 206) will nourish you for a full afternoon. If you feel you need more calories for lunch, simply add a high-quality protein source or a complex carbohydrate.

If you are rushed for lunch, it is best to have a shake as described in the "Breakfast" section. That way you will avoid creating the toxic breakdown products of undigested food eaten under stress.

Dinner

Dinner is often the most relaxed meal of the day—a time when you can slow down and really enjoy what you are eating. Try any of the options mentioned for lunch.

Here is an opportunity to make up for what may have been lacking in your food choices during the day. Think about what you have eaten so far. Have you taken in your thirty to sixty grams of fiber for optimal health? If not, you may choose to eat a lot of vegetables for dinner and a high-fiber dessert such as Antioxidant Fruit Salad (page 196), Better Than Chocolate Pudding (page 210), Silly Pudding (page 213), or Mild Laxative Treats (page 214). Did you take in your appropriate amount of omega-3 fatty acids as described in Chapter 3? If not, have one of the dressings mentioned above on your salad, grains, or vegetables, eat fish for dinner, or at least take one or two DHA capsules (depending on your weight and what you have already taken in during the day) to allow your nervous system to recharge while you sleep.

If you have not had enough pure water during the day (at least thirty-two ounces) drink some as soon as you get home. If you drink it too close to bedtime, you may have to make unexpected trips to the bathroom when you would be better off dreaming.

For your intestinal health, in addition to the fiber, EFAs, and water, have you had your probiotics? Be sure to eat one of the following: yogurt, kefir, Probioplex Intensive Care, or Ultra Flora Plus.

If you have fulfilled all of these recommendations, you can go to bed knowing you have done the best you could do for yourself this day nutritionally. If you did not, then you have the option of making healthier choices tomorrow.

Bon appétit!

CHAPTER 14

SUPPLEMENTS TO SUPPORT CLEANSING

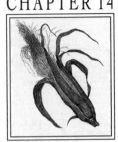

DETOXIFICATION TEA

If you prefer doing a mild cleanse and finding your nutrients in herbal teas, I recommend Detoxification Tea from Mountain Wild Herbals. The ingredients are red clover, horsetail, nettles, alfalfa, oat straw, licorice, and rose hips. These herbs are all grown organically, dried fresh, and sent to you (see Appendix 1 for ordering information). Detoxification Tea is supportive to the acid/base balance. It is gently alkalinizing, to neutralize the acid-inducing stress of our modern lives, and high in vitamins and minerals. (Its previous name was Daily Essentials, to acknowledge its use as a multivitamin and mineral support supplement.) The ingredients (in alphabetical order) contain the following nutritional factors:

> **Alfalfa:** potassium, magnesium, iron, manganese, copper, calcium, phosphorus, and vitamins A, C, D, E, K, B_1, B_{12}, and niacin

Horsetail: calcium, silica, bioflavonoids, iron, magnesium

Licorice: phosphorus, iron, magnesium

Nettles: calcium, phosphorus, potassium, iron, silica, copper, sulfur, and vitamins A, C, D, and K

Oat straw: magnesium, steroidal saponins (stabilize blood sugar), and calcium (and synergistic minerals and vitamins that aid calcium absorption); reduces cholesterol and risk of heart disease; nourishes central nervous system

Red clover: vitamins B-complex and C, calcium

Rose hips: vitamin C

In tea form, the nutrients are easy to assimilate because they are more like a food. They smell delicious and are easy to make. In my office, we brew up a pot in the morning and keep it out in a thermal teapot for our staff, clients, and patients.

PROBIOTIC FORMULAS

Probiotics are a class of nutrients that supply and encourage health-promoting bacteria in your intestines. They include, but are not limited to, mothers' milk, fiber acidophilus, bifido-bacteria, fructooligosaccharides (FOS), and inulin, which can be found in Kalenite (a component of dandelion) and Ultra Clear Sustain. As you have learned in previous chapters, healthy intestines support your good health by promoting the formation of B-vitamins, immune boosters, and anticarcinogenic substances. You may use probiotics every day, not only when you cleanse but to improve your health and well-being.

When choosing a probiotic formula to recommend to my patients, I considered four factors:

1. Stomach acid and bile resistance: will the friendly bacteria live through the digestive process to colonize in your bowel?
2. Research indicates that the NCFM (North Carolina Food and Microbiology) strain of acidophilus survives the digestive process and then attaches itself to the intestinal wall where it grows. Metagenics/Ethical Nutrients holds the exclusive right to use the NCFM strain.
3. Refrigeration: The beneficial bugs need a cool environment in the outside world to stay alive. If the product is on the shelf in the health food store or was not shipped in a refrigerated package, it is probably useless.
4. Independent laboratory assays: Each batch of Metagenics probiotic formulas has been assayed by a lab independent of Metagenics to assure the quantity and viability of the friendly bacteria that they claim are in the bottle.

A study by Vicki L. Hughes, M.T., and Sharon L. Hilier, Ph.D., of the Department of Obstetrics and Gynecology, University of Washington, Seattle, looked at the effect of acidophilus products on vaginitis, which causes itching and discharge from the vagina. As a preliminary step, they analyzed approximately twenty different acidophilus products to find the best one to use in their study. Only one product had any viable, living acidophilus in it. The rest of the products not only did not have the "good guys" in the bottle, they included pathogenic or disease-producing bacteria. Although the one product contained live acidophilus cultures, we do not know if it could hold up to the rigorous standards required of the Metagenics product, Ultra Flora Plus, that I recommend. Ultra Flora Plus is available at nutritionally minded doctors' offices, in regular and dairy-free forms (see Appendix 1).

Cultured milk products such as yogurt may also contain beneficial live cultures of what we affectionately call in our office "bif and doph"—the friendly bacteria. However, because of the problem with Bovine Somatotropic Hormone (BSH—a potential carcinogen; see Chapter 4) being used by commercial dairies to increase their milk yields, I recommend getting yogurt made from the milk of organically raised cows. You can generally find organically made yogurt in your health food store. If that is not possible, the next best choice is non-fat yogurt from your supermarket; hormone residue lives in the fat portion of milk products, so by eliminating the fat you are better protected. Here is another label reading opportunity: make sure the label states that the product contains live cultures. Some companies heat yogurt after it is packed, which destroys our little friends.

Another probiotic formula, Probioplex Intensive Care by Metagenics, combines a number of nutritional components that nourish friendly bacteria and obliterate harmful microbes. Nourishment is provided from FOS (discussed at length in Chapter 9), maltodexetrin, and lecithin. A team of nutrients: concentrated activated globulin whey, lactoferrin, and lactoperoxidase, coat, starve, and kill the "bad guys." In a process called opsonization, the activated globulin coats the pathogens and alerts your immune system cells to their presence. Lactoferrin binds to iron in the colon, a food source for pathogenic microorganisms depriving them of nourishment (your body receives all the iron it needs by absorption higher up in your small intestines). Finally, lactoperoxidase kills the "bad guys" by damaging their cell walls. This team of nutrients acts selectively against harmful microbes and for the health and proliferation of the "good guys." Dairy sensitive people may not be able to tolerate this product (for more information see Appendix 1).

FREE RADICALS AND OXIDATIVE STRESS

Free radicals are highly reactive molecules, originating from internal and external pollution, that can cause tissue damage by reacting with fatty acids in your cell membranes, portions of your DNA, and critical bonds in your protein structures (joints, muscles, organs, glands, and so on). To visualize the damage that free radicals can do, think about what exposure to air does to a cut apple or to untreated metal: apples turn brown and taste bad, and metal rusts. Free radicals have been implicated in the development of more than fifty diseases, including allergies, fibromyalgia, chronic fatigue, arthritis and other inflammatory diseases, neurological diseases, kidney disease, cataracts, bowel disease, lung dysfunction, drug reactions, skin problems, and aging. Heart disease and cancer are strongly associated with free-radical damage. More and more studies are linking low dietary intake of antioxidants to an increased risk of heart disease. Antioxidants are nutrients that bind to toxins and biochemically alter their chemical structure. Conversely, a reduction of cancer risk is associated with diets high in antioxidants such as vitamin C. Free radicals cause damage to your cells resulting in internal pollution in your body.

Solutions to Free Radical Stress

Saturate your environment with negative ions, which help trap positively charged pollution particles. You can purchase negative-ion generators, but they tend to make a big black spot on surfaces near where they do their work because they're attracting soot and pollution particles. Some newer models have a foam collar that is intended to catch the pollution particles so that they don't collect on your walls and furniture, but they are not completely effective.

You can also get negative ions for free; they are present in the mist of running water, among other things. A friend in chiropractic school had a solution for whatever ailed you: take a shower. Sometimes she took three showers a day. Once I learned about the high concentration of negative ions in shower spray, I had a better understanding of her panacea. A shower is especially good if you have a water filter in place (see Appendix 1 for information on where you can find a water filter).

Other suggestions for increasing your "happy particle" stream include taking a walk at night since negative ions are more highly concentrated in the night air, spending time with plants (pointed plant leaves concentrate negative ions), and performing yogic breathing exercises. To do the latter, breathe through one nostril at a time by closing down the other nostril with your thumb or middle finger.

Oxidative Stress

Oxidative stress is the cellular damage caused by free radicals. Antioxidant supplements and antioxidant foods trap these free radicals, protecting your cells and improving the outcome of your cleansing programs (for more on antioxidant foods see Chapter 14). Are you at risk for oxidative stress? See the Oxidative Stress Questionnaire in Appendix 4 to find out. A "yes" to any of these questions may mean that you are not meeting your antioxidant needs and thus are vulnerable to the damage that free radicals can cause. If you do have oxidative stress, see Appendix 1 for the types of nutrients that quench free radicals.

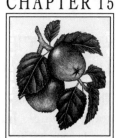

CHAPTER 15

PRACTICES THAT COMPLEMENT CLEANSING

When embarking on an internal cleansing program, there are several techniques that can complement and enhance the process. They will encourage a more active cleansing and prevent any possibility of severe cleansing reactions. I feel that the most important of these techniques are: conscious relaxation, drinking water, exercise, skin brushing, and supplementing your diet with aloe vera, bentonite, and the probiotics we discussed in Chapters 13 and 14.

We have seen that the world in which we live places an amazing burden on the natural cleansing systems of our bodies. If you do not assist your cleansing systems in removing the waste your cells are swimming in every day, you may be subject to degenerative diseases that could rob you of a happy, healthy life. But as you incorporate cleansing practices into your lifestyle, you will receive many other benefits of good health.

EVALUATE THE HEALTH IMPACT OF YOUR PRIORITIES

The Greek philosopher Epictetus said, "Men are disturbed not by things, but by the view they take of them." Our minds can be our greatest ally, but also our greatest enemy. It is important to determine what role your thoughts, emotions, and beliefs actually play with respect to your health.

There are no shortcuts to health any more than there are to raising healthy crops or animals. To be in good health, you must first be clear about how much you value your health. Then you must live a life of integrity in alignment with the timeless, unchanging laws and principles that govern health. A beneficial exercise is to pause and write down what you value in life and what those things you value mean to you. Take your time. Perhaps revisit what you have written a day or two later. Are you making time for what you value in your life? If not, you will benefit by spending half an hour a week to shape your schedule around what is important before you get swallowed by the river of life. Steven Covey's *First Things First* (Simon & Schuster, 1994) is a good guide to life management.

LOSE TOXIC-LADEN FAT

One of the most common benefits reported by those who have done internal cleansing is that they seem to lose weight without even trying. When you lose weight, you are losing fat if you follow a careful cleansing program such as I've described. As you have read, fat is the storage place for toxins in your body. When you lose fat, you are helping to decrease your toxic load. Much of the weight loss comes from the stomach and waistline, where a distended colon has given the appearance of fat. Many people who have dieted for years, and have lost weight in all portions of their bodies except the stubborn stomach region, find that these protrusions disappear through cleansing. If you have been unable to lose that thick area around your middle, it may not be due solely to overeating as much as to a desperate need to cleanse your intestines.

In addition, cleansing the intestinal tract will enable your body's systems to work more efficiently so that you will absorb more nutrients from the foods that you eat. Many times, people eat too much because their body is not being nutritionally satisfied from the foods they eat. This is caused not only by eating the wrong foods but also by a sluggish, blocked system that is unable to absorb nutrients. Both a high-fiber diet and a thorough cleansing will greatly enhance nutrient absorption and reduce the tendency to be addicted to foods that have no nutritional value.

Reducing the volume of carbohydrates that you eat in the form of grains, bread, pasta, crackers, waffles, pancakes, and so on may also help you get rid of unwanted fat. A long-term patient of mine has been trying to lose that last five pounds ever since she had her children, more than twenty years ago, but whatever she tried failed. Finally, she took my advice and eliminated almost all grains and grain products from her diet. She is now happy to show me her flat stomach and celebrate losing those last five pounds.

EXERCISE TO STIMULATE THE CLEANSING PROCESS

In addition to a proper diet, the value of regular exercise cannot be overstated. Remember how toxins are primarily stored in the fatty tissue of your body? By mobilizing this toxic fat through exercise, deep breathing, sweating, and drinking lots of water, you will rid your body of this reservoir of harmful substances. Our bodies are designed for movement, and in our increasingly sedentary lives it is most important to incorporate some consistent physical activity into your schedule. If you are following the type of diet recommended in previous chapters—high in fruits and vegetables, low in animal fats, and with the proper proportions of essential fatty acids and healthy protein—you will be able to reduce the nonbeneficial fat stored in your cells to recreate a healthier you with added exercise.

First, let's take a look at the benefits of exercise, then we will examine some ways to fit more activity into your busy schedule.

1. Exercise strengthens and tones the muscles of the body, including those in your gastrointestinal tract. It helps to stimulate a sluggish bowel. If you are prone to constipation, exercise will help increase the activity of your bowel, making you a much more efficient eliminator of metabolic waste products.

2. Exercise increases circulation and perspiration. Your skin is your largest organ of elimination. When you sweat, toxins that are circulating in your blood and lymph and stored in the subcutaneous layers of your skin are released through your pores, assisting your body's cleansing process and strengthening your immune system.

3. Exercise strengthens your lungs' ability to transport oxygen to your heart and to carry carbon dioxide and waste away from it.

4. Exercise increases lymphatic circulation, which supports the excretion of waste from your cells.

5. A regular exercise program greatly reduces the effects of stress and increases self-esteem. Chemicals of stress that build up in your system can be metabolized more efficiently when you exercise. Have you ever noticed how much better you feel after taking a walk if something is troubling you? Part of the transformation comes from the breakdown of stress hormones that have stayed lodged in your nervous system just waiting for release.

6. Exercise raises your metabolic rate to more efficiently utilize the calories you take in, especially if you exercise within one half-hour of eating.

7. Consistently following an exercise program makes you feel more balanced, healthier, stronger, and more self-confident.

Regular exercise strengthens all of your body's systems, enabling you to function optimally. The natural cleansing and elimination systems that are so valuable to you in preventing the build up of toxic waste will be made stronger and more efficient by physical activity. Steven Blair, M.D., has this to say about exercise in his book, *Living with Exercise* (American Health Publishing Co., 1991): "A good exercise prescription for the thirty to fifty million mostly sedentary and unfit Americans is 'turn off the television, get off your fanny, go out the door, and move around a bit.' We have learned from research that it often doesn't matter what you do. Any activity that increases your metabolic rate and burns more calories provides benefits." Whether you choose an aerobic activity (one that raises your heart rate significantly) or a series of stretching exercises, what is most important is consistency. It is said that if you maintain an exercise program for six months, it will become a healthy habit for life. Even a brisk walk taken for ten minutes daily will benefit you in many ways. Here's a wonderful quote about exercise from Edward Stanley, the Earl of Derby, in 1873: "Those who think they have not time for bodily exercise will sooner or later have to find time for illness."

It is never too late to begin an exercise program. William Evans, Ph.D., Chief of the Human Physiology Laboratory at Tufts University, Human Nutrition Research Center on Aging, has witnessed a ninety-year-old patient become stronger than a fifty-year-old through consistent exercise. The center's oldest exerciser is 100 years of age. One of my fifty-five-year-old male patients belongs to a softball team called the "Seniors." Their age range is from fifty to seventy. When you get older than seventy in their league, you join the "Creakers," who play on a team of men from seventy to ninety years of age.

How do you fit more activity into a busy but largely sedentary lifestyle? You have heard this before: park your car a block away from where you are going so that you get more leg work on your way to and from your errands. If you live in an area with public transportation, consider taking it once in a while; generally there is some extra walking getting back and forth between stations or bus stops. Take the stairs instead of the elevator, if not the whole way at least for a landing or two. Stand up when you are talking on the telephone; it will make your voice stronger and give you the opportunity to stretch or move your legs. To multiply the effect on your metabolic activity, gently march or step in place while talking.

While standing, you might also take the opportunity to do some pliés (pronounced 'plea-ayz'), as they are called in the dance world: keeping your back straight, place your feet a comfortable distance apart, bend your knees and lower your torso straight down a comfortable distance, then rise up by straightening your legs, and repeat. This exercise has the benefit of increasing your circulation. I remember waiting at 7:00 A.M. for my chiropractic licensing board exam to begin. A friend and I were taking the boards at the same time. We had gotten lost on the way to the exam, so we were pretty stressed out. When the examiners came parading past, I started to feel faint. Pliés saved me from passing out that day. Bending my knees and straightening them helped to get more blood moving up into my head. Pliés can even boost your performance on the job by helping you think more clearly in place of that afternoon cup of toxic coffee.

If you have stairs at home, try walking up and down them a couple of times after eating; it will help combat that after-meal brain fog that too often brings your energy down. Or just try dancing. One of my favorite ways to exercise is to put on James Brown's "Gravity" CD and let loose! Even if you don't have music, you can make music with the rhythmic movement of your body. Here's a chance to let the kid in you out and have more fun—a great antidote for the complexity and seriousness of life. I have a lot of fun standing outside my car and stretching at gas stations when my tank is filling. Sometimes I even use the paper receptacles to stretch out my hamstrings. (Be sure to watch out for car movement while engaging in your gas-station stretch routine.) While on an airplane, I always go to the open area adjacent to the movie screen and do some stretching. That raises some eyebrows, but I also notice that my stretching sets an example for other people to get off their duffs to stretch or just walk around. Some don't bother to get up, but stretch in their seats anyway.

One of my dear friends has lived for a couple of years in China. She reports that people are much more active there. They do Tai Chi in the parks, massage reflex points on their bodies and faces, and walk and ride bicycles much more than we do in this country. Why not be the first to start a revolution in your office, home, or town? Bob Anderson has some great books on stretching. He has gone so far as to make up a sheet of exercises that can be done right at your desk to ease the monotony of minuscule motions that one performs while in an office setting. (For more information, see Appendix 1.)

Conversely, if you are the kind of person who does a lot of physical work on the job, you probably need to stretch more than you need to strengthen your muscles. Your local college or YMCA/YWCA probably has some stretch or yoga classes that would benefit you—or buy one of the many stretching videos that are on the market and use it.

Therein lies the key, doesn't it? Make the time to just do it! Working with your schedule is essential here. Steven Covey encourages us to decide what we value in our lives and then to make time for what we value by putting those things into our schedule before anything else. Did you know that in our country the most successful people and businesses spend up to sixty percent of their time planning? Plan for success this time. Either make a time in your day that is sacred—that you devote to taking good care of yourself with some type of movement—or just commit to being more active in general. Write down your successes in the area of increased movement or exercise, and celebrate. You can do it!

TAKE A BATH AND SWEAT IT OUT

If you are unable to exercise to a level that makes you sweat, you can enjoy the benefits of sweating by taking a sauna, steam bath, hot tub, or hot bath. One of my best suggestions for my patients that are sore or achy and complaining of stiff muscles as a result of toxic build up is to take a bath with Epsom salts. Magnesium salts are the main ingredient of Epsom salts. Magnesium is great for relaxing tight, sore, and tired muscles. It helps carry calcium into your muscle cells to relax them and helps your cells to get rid of toxins. (You may also take a magnesium supplement to relax your muscles if you cannot take baths. Magnesium glycinate is preferred because it is gentle to your digestive tract. Other forms of magnesium can cause diarrhea. Magnesium Glycinate is made and distributed by Metagenics and is available through doctor's offices.) Soaking in hot water, in and of itself, has a relaxing effect on your body, mind, and soul, but you can enhance that effect by putting essential oils into your bath. Only a little is needed, because the oil will disperse in the water. Pine is said to help sore muscles and joints, and lavender is said to soothe and calm your nervous system. If you stay in the room while the tub fills, you will have the added benefit of a negative ion bath.

BREATHE DEEPLY TO REPLACE BAD AIR WITH GOOD

Air is our first necessity for continued life. Some accomplished yogis and pearl divers are able to hold their breath or suspend overt signs of breathing for extended periods of time; however, the average human has no such skills. The human brain dies after being deprived of oxygen for one to two minutes.

There are ways to expand your breathing repertoire that will increase your health. Deep breathing helps exchange the "good" air for the "bad" air. Some benefits of deep breathing are:

- The relaxation response is enhanced when you are breathing deeply. When you are more relaxed, your body works better and life seems to go better, too. Be careful, however: you may hyperventilate and feel dizzy if you neglect to expand your whole torso all the way down to your pubic bone with each breath.
- Deep breathing can help normalize the pH in your body and support metabolic function. It helps calm the spirit and soothe the soul. It will quickly take you out of a sympathetic nervous system alarm state and reduce the stress you are feeling in the moment.
- Deep breathing may help prevent lung cancer. The apex, or top part, of the lungs that sits above your collarbone is the most common site of lung cancer. Some lung cancer begins here perhaps because people usually breathe shallow breaths that don't expand this area. Since air is not exchanged there, it becomes a collection spot for particulate matter (such as pollution) from the air. Think of a closet or drawer that you don't go into often but that is exposed to air from the outside world: it stays shut up and collects dust. The same thing can happen with your upper lungs.

There are many excellent resources in the area of breath work: yoga classes often help you focus on breathing techniques, guided relaxation audio tapes direct you to breathe deeply and slowly, and there are a number of books on the topic. (See Appendix 1 for more information.)

REDUCE TOXINS WITH CHIROPRACTIC CARE

Injury from microtrauma, for example, working at your computer for long hours or macrotrauma such as a fall or auto accident (see Chapter 1, "Structural Stress") cause an accumulation of tissue damaging toxins in your body. Studies done around the world have shown the benefits of chiropractic care in reducing or eliminating these toxic by-products of injury that lead to stiffness and pain. In New Zealand and Canada, government economists who studied the issue recommended that people with back pain see a chiropractor first so that they would be able to go back to work faster and save their governments millions of dollars.

But, as before, the most important criterion in *Internal Cleansing* is the response of you, the public. And that information is available in terms of patient satisfaction. Several studies have shown that patients are more satisfied with chiropractic care than with medical care. And what about our senior citizens? If something can help our grandparents and aging relatives enjoy a greater level of health and vitality, would it be worth checking out for yourself? *Topics in Clinical Chiropractic* published a study which showed that elderly chiropractic patients reported better overall health, had fewer chronic conditions, spent fewer days in nursing homes and hospitals, were more mobile in their communities, and were more likely to report strenuous levels of exercise than nonchiropractic patients. In short, they were less toxic than those not receiving chiropractic adjustments. In fact, eighty-seven percent of chiropractic patients described their health status as good to excellent, compared to sixty-eight percent of nonchiropractic patients.

Chiropractic just became a centenarian itself. We celebrated our 100th anniversary in September of 1996. Chiropractic comprises many techniques, but all of them begin with a perspective of removing the interference in your nervous system to allow your internal healing abilities to shine bright. One recent study that I particularly love describes the effect of chiropractic adjustments on the immune system. The study was performed at the National College of Chiropractic, and it measured white blood cell (WBC) activity pre- and post-adjustment. When WBCs go into action to defend you against foreign invaders, they increase their oxygen uptake as measured by an increase in luminescence in the blood sample. What this means is that chiropractic adjustments help to turn on your healing light.

Brush Your Skin

The value of dry skin brushing has been known for centuries. The Finns and Russians used birch twigs to open their pores and stimulate circulation before a steam bath or sauna. The Turks used coarse towels to rub dead skin off their body before and after the bath.

As the largest eliminative organ, the skin plays a vital role in ridding your body of the toxins and impurities that are potential sources of illness. It has been estimated that the skin eliminates over one pound of waste per day. For this reason, daily skin brushing goes hand in hand with an internal cleansing program.

Dry skin brushing is one of the best ways to cleanse the skin without removing the protective mantle of acid and oils. Daily skin brushing removes the top layer of dead skin with its buildup of dirt and acid and deeply cleanses your pores.

Skin brushing is also one of the most powerful ways to cleanse your lymphatic system. Waste material is carried away from the cells by the blood and the lymph. Skin brushing stimulates the release of this material from the cells near the surface of your skin.

In addition, dry skin brushing stimulates the sweat glands and increases blood circulation to underlying organs and tissues of the body. These days, a sedentary lifestyle, a general lack of exercise, and the use of antiperspirants keep people from perspiring enough. As a result, toxins and metabolic waste products become trapped in the body instead of being released through sweat. Skin brushing opens up the pores, allowing your body to breathe and thus enhancing proper function of your organs.

Skin brushing has also been a beauty aid of men and women for ages Removing the top layer of dead skin and stimulating blood circulation are essential for maintaining youthful, glowing, and supple skin. Loss of excess weight and cellulite is an added benefit reported by a beauty salon owner in Santa Barbara, California: "I use skin brushing as part of my weight-loss and body shaping program. Skin brushing increases circulation, which helps to draw out the stored waste and toxins which often result in cellulite buildup. People tend to lose weight faster and more evenly over the entire body when skin brushing is included in their weight loss program."

How to Skin Brush

First, acquire an all-natural-vegetable-fiber brush from your health food store (synthetic fibers will irritate your skin). A long handle is helpful for reaching your back and the entire surface of your body.

The best time to brush is before taking a shower or bath. Brushing dry skin is important, as sagging may occur if your skin or the brush is wet. Begin by brushing with one-stroke movements. Brush from the outermost points—your feet and hands—toward the center of your body. Brush across your upper back and down the front and back of your torso. Cover the entire surface of the skin only once. A slight flush is normal due to increased circulation, but if your skin turns red you may be brushing too hard.

For your face, use a softer brush or leave it alone since the blood vessels are nearer the surface of your skin and can be broken if brushed too hard. If you do brush your face, begin in the center and stroke outward, then up the sides of your face and neck.

The total process takes only about three minutes. When you are finished, jump into your bath or shower and enjoy. You will feel an invigorating, tingling sensation over your entire body.

RELAX AND REST TO SUPPORT YOUR CLEANSING

As we have discussed, negative thoughts, moods, and emotions create toxins within your body and excess stress promotes an overgrowth of pathogenic microorganisms with their subsequent build up of toxic by-products in your intestines. Creating "healing intervals," times in which you "stop to smell the roses" so to speak, are vital to your ability to cleanse and heal. William Penn, founder of the state of Pennsylvania, said, "True silence is the rest of the mind; it is to the spirit what sleep is to the body: nourishment and refreshment." In questionnaires I use with my patients, I ask them about the amount of time they spend resting during their day and how they spend their "resting" time. Often they cite watching TV as their rest time. But television watching is not the kind of healing, restorative relaxation to which we are referring.

My favorite definitions of "rest" from Webster's Dictionary are "peace of mind or spirit" and "to be free from anxiety or disturbance." Because we are all unique individuals, we will find our peace of mind and freedom from anxiety in different ways. Currently, I most enjoy sitting on the edge of my bed, closing my eyes, placing a smile on my face, and focusing on a state of joy. When my attention drifts, I gently bring my focus back to the state of bliss that awaits me. Enjoying the beauty of nature also quickly restores my soul. When I was twenty-two, sitting calmly made me feel agitated, so I took "LSD" (a "long slow distance" run) or I did *katas* that I had learned in my karate classes. Here are some other recommendations for rest:

- take a bath or soak in a hot tub
- smile and allow the smile to wash over your entire face and body (I will explain this technique in further detail later in this chapter)
- take a deep breath
- adopt an attitude of gratitude — pause for a moment to reflect on what you have to be grateful for in your life
- smell a fragrant flower

- hum or sing a song in your shower or in your car where no one else is listening—or if you have a good voice let others enjoy your singing out loud
- stretch your arms and legs
- scrunch up your face and wiggle your mouth around, then take a deep breath and sigh
- try to wiggle your ears
- dance or sway to music
- laugh for no reason

Norman Cousins, who overcame a life-threatening disease by watching Marx Brothers movies and taking lots of vitamin C, says, "Laughter is inner jogging." The possibilities are endless. Here's something I read about in my Sunday paper: pet a chicken. The December 1, 1996, issue of *The San Francisco Examiner* had this headline: "Chickens' new job: Lifting seniors' spirits: Saved from frying pan, birds become traveling therapists." Darrian Lundy of Green Acres farms brings her two chickens, Chickadee and Spock, to a center for older folks. "It gets people talking who haven't talked all week and generally raises their spirits," she said.

Using self-help techniques can enhance the quality of your health and your life. Your thoughts and emotions are energetic and biochemical. They have a significant impact on your health and on your relationships with others. If you dwell on worry and fear because of a past pain you experienced in some part of your body, heart, or mind, you will reinforce your pain. If you do nothing to transform that worry and fear, your being will store that negativity, and you may end up with or aggravate a degenerative condition. Choose to send love and happiness to your entire being—mind, body, and soul—and you will enjoy greater health.

Pursuing health will be joyous work if you focus your awareness and heart on the task.

Why don't you take a moment now to jot down some ways of relaxing that you would enjoy? Pull your list out and try one the next time you are exceeding your health limits. Here's some advice from Leonardo da Vinci, painter, architect, and inventor: "Every now and then go away, even briefly; have a little relaxation, for when you come back to your work your judgment will be surer; since to remain constantly at work will cause you to loose power. . . ."

During a cleanse, when you feel like resting, take a few minutes out for a nap or meditation and pause to appreciate the good that is being accomplished by the release of toxins. Buckminster Fuller knew the value of the semiconscious resting place between sleep and wakefulness. He developed a method to capitalize on this most creative, insightful time. His technique was to lean back in a high-back leather chair so that his head was supported, place a couple of small balls in his hand, and drift off as deeply and quickly as he could. If he fell asleep, the muscles of his hand would relax and the balls would fall and wake him instantly. As he heard the noise of the balls hitting the floor, he awakened rejuvenated and refreshed. Even closing your eyes, leaning back, and taking a deep breath can give you an instantaneous recharge.

Frequently during the day, humans build up tension all through their bodies. Muscle tension creates metabolic waste products that further irritate your musculoskeletal system and your subconscious. Taking a few minutes to focus on relaxing that tension will enable you to sustain a higher energy level and feel better during your busy schedule. Try one of these exercises next time you need a break:

NECK ROLL/SHOULDER LIFTS   Sitting or standing, close your eyes and take a deep breath. Drop your head forward, then slowly rotate it to the side, then lift your chin and stretch your head up and slightly to the back if comfortable, and then roll down to the other side. Continue in a circle three times in each direction. Now lift both shoulders up toward your ears, squeeze tight, flushing out all of your neck and shoulder tension, hold for a moment, and release. Coordinating your breathing will amplify the benefits: inhale as you draw your shoulders up and squeeze; exhale as you release. Repeat approximately eight times.

PROGRESSIVE RELAXATION   If you can lie down for a few moments, or at least rest back with your head supported, try this one. Beginning with your feet and working up your body, tighten each area of your body, one part at a time, to its maximum degree of tension. Now let go, either quickly and completely or slowly and gently, and wait a few seconds, enjoying the new sense of relaxation in that part of you. When you have tensed and relaxed each part of your body, tense and release your entire body and then rest in this state of tension-free bliss. You can pop the "Journey to Health" tape into your cassette player to guide you through this process (see Appendix 1 for ordering information).

SELF-APPROVAL   As I mentioned in the Introduction, our mind can be our greatest enemy, but also our strongest ally. We have a tendency to judge ourselves harshly and to drive ourselves to some distant ideal of perfection. This creates a state of mind that says we never have enough and we are never good enough. Stop a moment and feel how your body feels when you judge yourself. It doesn't feel good, does it? Now change that feeling to one of love, approval, and appreciation for the great person you are and for the wonderful things you do. Now how do you feel? You can take this positive feeling and direct it inward to restore and revitalize your health.

SLEEP   When doing your cleansing program, you may need more sleep than at other times, especially during the first few days. Often I think that the psychological component of changing habit patterns and wrestling with your mind to accomplish this wears you out, but there are also good physiological reasons for needing more rest. Your body is busy eliminating toxins and waste that has been housed in your tissues for years. Resting allows your body to concentrate its energy on this cleansing process. To get a more restful night's sleep, try stretching before you get into bed, or do the Progressive Relaxation technique described a few paragraphs earlier.

LET THE INNER SMILE TRANSFORM YOU

From the ancient Taoist system of healing comes a simple practice called "The Inner Smile." Smiling into your abdomen and into the rest of your body is one of the quickest and most economical ways to change your mood and your physical state.

Master Mantak Chia, Director of the Healing Tao and Tao Garden and author of numerous books on healing and meditation practices, teaches the "Inner Smile," a powerful tool for self-healing. Chia says, "Smiling to yourself is like basking in love; you become your own best friend!"

Take a few moments and try this simple meditation. It will guide you through a process of smiling into every cell of your body for rejuvenation and healing. (For an audio-cassette of this relaxing and healing meditation, see Appendix 1.)

Wear comfortable clothing and sit relaxed in a chair. You can also try this practice lying down, but the danger is that you will fall asleep from becoming so relaxed. Place your hands comfortably in your lap, your right palm on top of your left. Breathe easily from your abdomen and gently close your eyes. Imagine that you are with someone you love or in a beautiful place in which you feel peace and joy. Picture yourself smiling, lift up the corners of your mouth, and feel the smiling energy in your eyes, too. Allow this energy to begin to soak into your body through a point between your eyebrows or on the top of your head. One of my students felt best imagining the energy flowing into his heart. Feel the energy flow like a waterfall down your face, into your eyes, relaxing your jaw and face muscles. Everywhere the smile touches, you feel more relaxed and rejuvenated, more alive.

Let the smiling energy flow into your throat and neck now, moving into and filling your heart. As your heart fills with the loving smile, thank your heart for working day and night to pump your blood, carrying nutrients and sweeping away waste from every tissue, organ, gland, and cell. Smile into your heart until your heart smiles back at you. Now let the smile spread out to both sides into your lungs. Thank your lungs for supplying life-giving air to all the parts of your body. Let the smile fill your entire lungs all the way up to and above your collarbones. Now, gently flowing down your body like a warm and soothing waterfall, smile into your liver, kidneys, spleen, intestines, bladder, genitals, spine, muscles, tendons, ligaments, bones, nerves, lymphatic system, skin, fatty tissue, hair, nails, and every cell. Smile into all of these areas until they smile back at you, and thank them for the tireless work they do to keep you alive and thriving. Enjoy the relaxed, tingling, alive, and excited feeling that all of you now feel from being touched by the smile—your smile.

When you have filled yourself and absorbed all of the goodness from your smile, bring your attention to your navel. Imagine that you have a ball or a treasure chest directly behind your belly button. Allow the excess bounty of the smiling energy to collect inside that place.

End your Inner Smile session by imaging a spiral at your naval, first in one direction then the other, to lock the bounty away until you need it. If you start to feel run down during the day, bring your attention to the magic ball or treasure chest just inside your body behind your navel and draw out some smiling treasure to restore your health and vitality.

You can take a half an hour or just a few seconds to enjoy the benefits of the Inner Smile. Why don't you pause for just a moment and lift up the corners of your mouth with a smile and feel your eyes smiling too. Let that smile wash over your entire body, mind, and soul. Inhale and feel it being absorbed into all of your tissues. It's as simple as that. Isn't that a great way to bring you back to what is important? Do you feel more centered and ready to go forth with your life? Can you imagine stringing a few of those moments together in your day? How would it feel if you were able to stay in this smiling state for an hour, or for a day?

For those of you who are more skeptical, just the thought of reaching inside your belly for treasure to enliven your day might give you a chuckle and help to change your state toward the better. There is scientific, measurable evidence that your physiological state changes because of a shift in your hormones when you smile. When you smile, not only does "the whole world smile with you," but smiling hormones are produced and released into your bloodstream. Hormones have powerful effects on your mood, thoughts, and behavior.

When people are depressed, their immune system is compromised. I am reminded of a "Peanuts" cartoon in which Charlie Brown is talking to a friend. He has his head dropped forward, slumped onto his chest, and he says, "This is my depressed stance. When you're depressed, it makes a lot of difference how you stand. . . . The worst thing you can do is straightening up and holding your head high because then you'll start to feel better. . . . If you're going to get any joy out of being depressed, you've got to stand like this." Smiling and standing up straight, with your head held high, allows you to lighten up and appreciate the good things in life instead of filling your cells with the toxic chemistry of negative thoughts and feelings.

CONCLUSION

Allopathic medicine works on a model of removing symptoms. If you have a headache, a fever, diarrhea, constipation, irregular heart beat, or high blood pressure, for instance, you are given a drug to stop the unpleasant manifestation of your internal disorder. If you have a growth, polyp, tumor, congested gallbladder, or damaged intestinal tract, it will be cut out without a thought as to why the problem has occurred. Instead, we should be asking questions: What is behind all of this dysfunction and disease? What is the fundamental reason that we lose our health and become sick?

As you have learned by reading this book, our environment plays a major role in the state of our health. Yet human beings have been in challenging or toxic situations since time immemorial, and some have the amazing ability to thrive as demonstrated by human achievement as described in the following stories.

We hear of mothers who lift automobiles off their children who are pinned underneath. Thomas Edison tried over two thousand experiments before his invention, the light bulb, worked. A young reporter asked him how it felt to fail so many times. He said, "I never failed once. I invented the light bulb. It just happened to be a two-thousand-step process." Beethoven progressively lost his hearing. He was completely deaf by the age of forty-six, yet his greatest works were written in his later years. Franklin Roosevelt was paralyzed by polio at the age of thirty-nine, yet he went on to become one of America's most loved and influential presidents.

Wilma Rudolf was the twentieth of twenty-two children. Her survival was questionable right from birth. At age four, she became paralyzed in her left leg after a bout with double pneumonia and scarlet fever. At nine years of age, she took off her brace and began to walk. At thirteen she decided to become a runner. For the next few years, she finished last in every race she entered. After she eventually won a race her career skyrocketed, culminating in her winning three Gold Medals at the Olympics.

In *Spontaneous Remission: An Annotated Bibliography* by Brendan O'Regan and Caryle Hirshberg, you can read about a psychologist with rectal cancer. His doctor recommended immediate surgery. He refused any medical treatment, but sought the guidance of a therapist who taught meditation. Three hours of meditation every day reversed the debilitating complications of the rectal cancer, allowing him to return to his profession and continue with his favorite sport, hang gliding.

Do you remember the biblical story of Job? Job was a rich man with a loving wife and family until pestilence came upon him. He lost all of his material possessions. His neighbors and even his family turned their backs on him. He lost his health and still he would not despair; he continued to have faith. Finally all was restored.

There is within each of us a life force beyond what we eat, drink, or take in the form of pills that ensures our survival and gives us the ability to thrive. It cannot be measured by any of our scientific instruments, and doctors are not able to predict who will be able to mobilize this force to heal. What is evident is that those of us who feel loved and who focus on our health have a better-than-average chance.

I hope that you are now inspired and motivated to begin an internal cleansing program. Hundreds of thousands of people with a myriad of ailments have performed one form of cleansing or another over the millennia, and have benefited from the resulting renewed health and vitality. My own results and those of my clients and patients motivated me to share this information with you.

Never before have we been so in need of this knowledge. With the plethora of dangers that threaten our world today, it is easy to overlook the ills festering inside ourselves. As one woman said after completing her two-month cleansing program, "It's almost scary to see what you carry around inside, and it's a terrific feeling to know you got rid of that awful stuff." Other patients have said, "I began to feel better all over, and I have acquired a new energy," and, "It's like being reborn. I can't remember the last time I felt so good and had so much energy." There are many more testimonials from patients and clients who have had their lives changed by internal cleansing. From arthritis to allergies, whatever your problem, a good, safe cleansing program is sure to help. Your age or state of health doesn't matter. You can begin today to rebuild your own health.

Please do not postpone enjoying life until some future day when you are totally detoxified and have everything you could want in your life. Take action steps to minimize or eliminate the causes of your distress. Look for joy, peace, and happiness now. It may not be available in the outside world, but it is available every moment inside of you.

When the world deals you lemons, make lemonade. *Carpe diem!*

You may reach Dr. Linda Berry at:

1700 Solano Ave., Suite A
Berkeley, CA 94707
510-526-6657

or

723 Center Blvd.
Fairfax, CA 94930
415-456-1300

APPENDIX 1: RESOURCES AND PRODUCTS

GENERAL

Anatomy

If you desire further information on the location of your body parts, *The Anatomy Coloring Book* (Addison Wesley, 1993) by Wynn Kopit and Laurance M. Ellson is a great resource for learning more about your body. The material is presented in a simple, easy-to-understand format.

INTRODUCTION

Health Coach Information

To support your cleansing process, my recommendation is to seek out a Health Coach in your area. The collective purpose of Health Coach is to teach, inspire, and support people to improve the quality of their health by improving the quality of their living. Health Coaches are committed to enriching lives through education and natural therapies.

If you would like to learn more about the internal workings of the human body, I would refer you to some of the educational tools available within the Health Coach System. *Functional Dietetics* is the most comprehensive guide today on dietary habits with respect to health. Learn the fundamentals of nutrition, what constitutes a complete diet, what role digestion plays and how you can improve yours, what detoxification is, how you can change your health, what role food allergies or intolerances play and how you can identify them, the role your doctor can play with respect to your nutrition program, and perhaps most importantly, what foods enhance healing and what foods lead to disease.

In video format, Health Coach offers *The Disease/Toxicity Connection* and *Digestion, Detoxification, and Your Health*. These videos will show you why the fastest and surest way to detoxify your system is through improving the quality of your digestion. Dr. Percival states: "Understanding and implementing effective detoxification protocols may well be your most important step in regaining and rebuilding your health."

You may reach Health Coach by calling 800-463-2701 to locate a trained Health Coach professional in your area or to obtain educational materials.

CHAPTER 1: FOUR KINDS OF STRESS

Biochemical Stress

There is a newsletter called *The Wary Canary*, published by Suzanne and Ed Randegger. This is a gold mine of information for people who have a sensitivity to environmental toxics. The Randeggers also publish *Environ: A Magazine for Ecological Living & Health*. You can order these from: Wary Canary Press, P.O. Box 2204, Fort Collins, CO 80525. Telephone: 970-493-8089.

In Dallas, Texas, Dr. William Rea supervises cleansing programs using nutritional supplements, exercise, and sauna therapy at The Environmental Health Center. You may contact Dr. Rea's office by calling 214-368-4132.

Mental/Emotional Stress

Health Coach offers some excellent tools in this arena of healing. *The Mind-Body Connection* is a four-part video series and study guide that can help you approach your health and healing with renewed awareness and vitality by learning the action steps that leaders in the field of mind/body medicine are using to improve their clients' health.

The language you use can serve to support your well-being, but too often it undermines your dreams and your self-confidence. *Power Talking,* an eight-part audio series by George Walther, helps you transform your culturally entrenched negative and powerless language into a dynamic vocabulary that will fuel your success. These materials are available by calling Health Coach at 800-463-2701.

CHAPTER 2: HOW THE BODY PROCESSES FOOD AND TOXINS

Thyroid Blood Tests

For more in-depth information on thyroid blood tests, contact:

The Broda O. Barnes, M.D., Research Foundation, Inc., P. O. Box 98, Trumbull, CT 06611, 203-261-2101.

If you suspect a low-functioning thyroid, the Foundation can help you locate a doctor in your area who has been trained in recognizing and treating this hormone imbalance. Their doctors also work with other endocrine or hormonal problems besides thyroid challenges to help you to find a balance in your entire hormonal system.

There are many types of thyroid therapy. Metagenics makes a product called Energetics which supports thyroid function. It's available by calling 888-85-HEALTH.

Antibiotics and Ear Infections

Learn why antibiotics may not be the best course of therapy for chronic ear infections, and discover other options, by reading *Childhood Ear Infections* (Group West, 1990) by Dr. Michael Schmidt.

CHAPTER 3: NATURAL ELEMENTS OF A CLEAN BOWEL

Essential Fatty Acids

You can get flaxseed meal with a nutty rich flavor, and if you need inspiration on how to use it order a cookbook called *Flax for Life! 101 Delicious Recipes and Tips Featuring Fabulous Flax Oil* by Jade Beutler by calling 888-85-HEALTH.

Dr. Donald Rudin and Clara Felix have recently published *Omega 3 Oils to Improve Mental Health, Fight Degenerative Diseases and Extend Your Life* (Garden City Park, NY: Avery Publishing Group, 1996) — an update of their book *The Omega 3 Phenomenon* (NY: Rawson, 1987). It is a very valuable resource for the way fats affect your health and well-being.

You can research the processing of oils in more depth in *The Facts About Fats* by John Finnegan (Berkeley, CA: Elysian Arts Books, 1993), who made an exhaustive study of oil-processing plants, visited researchers, read numerous volumes, and reviewed hundreds of original research articles to bring you this valuable information.

If you can't get your children to eat fresh flaxseed oil, try Essential Balance Junior from Omega Nutrition (800-745-8580).

If that doesn't work, perhaps you can encourage them to take a capsule of DHA in a supplement called Neuromins, a vegetarian source of EFAs from Martek (800-662-6339). You may also contact Martek for a brochure about the value of EFAs in your infant's development by calling 800-522-5512. For more information see Appendix 2.

High-quality oils are available from few sources; contact Omega Nutrition (800-661-3529) and Barlean's (800-445-3529) for your best options.

Chapter 5: Household and Other Personal Toxins

Water Filtration

To purify the water you use for drinking and cooking, my recommendation is to purchase the Doulton filter, available for approximately $150 by calling 888-85-HEALTH.

To filter chlorine from your shower water, the Pure Water Store in Greenbrae, California, sells filters to fit shower heads for less than $50. They have national associates who can sell and service combination charcoal carbon/reverse osmosis filters to fit under your sink. You can reach them by calling 800-776-7654.

Minimizing Pesticides

McKenzie Rock Flour is derived from basalt and andesite rock deposits of the Cascade Mountains of Oregon. I interviewed the owner of Remineralization Products, Inc., Lee Poindexter, and am satisfied that this is a sustainable product that does no harm to the environment or wildlife. You can order rock flour from Dan Weber, an independent distributor of McKenzie Rock Flour, by calling 800-339-0141 or from Lee at 541-344-2524.

Diatomaceous earth and other natural insecticides are available from Organic Plus, Inc. (800-933-2278).

Gardens Alive! is a company dedicated to increasing fruit and vegetable yields and increasing the beauty of lawns and flowers by using natural compounds complementary to the earth. The intent is to allow nature to find its balance, but when it needs help, to gently intervene. The first line of defense is to feed your plants to keep them healthy and strong enough to deter pests and environmental stressors like frost. The second line of defense is natural pest predators such as lady bugs, green lacewings, and birds. Gardens Alive! sells lacewings and lady beetles, but not birds. The third stage is to create barriers or traps to cut down on pest damage. These run the gamut from electronic flea catchers to pheromone lures to attract pests that would otherwise destroy fruit crops, and super-light barrier cloths that allow sunlight in to the plants while keeping crop-destroying insects out. As a last resort, they recommend using pest-killing plant or mineral compounds that break down quickly and are not harmful to people or the planet. You may contact Gardens Alive! to request a product catalog by phone: 812-537-8650; fax: 812-537-5708; or mail: 5100 Schenley Place, Lawrenceburg, IL 47025.

Yale University offers yet another option: Change the nature of the typical suburban landscape. Their recommendations come in the form of a book called *Redesigning the American Lawn: A Search for Environmental Harmony* (New Haven,

MA, and London: Yale University Press, 1993) by F. Herbert Bormann, Diana Balmori, and Gordon T. Gebalbe.

Mercury Amalgam Fillings

If you are going to have your fillings removed and replaced with composite material, call Cascade Consultants in Portland, Oregon, at 800-489-8055. Dr. Paula Bickle of Cascade Consultants is conducting a multisite study on mercury amalgam fillings. She is training doctors and dentists all over the country to work together as a team to safely remove this toxic substance from our mouths and to chelate this dangerous heavy metal from tissues in which it has been stored in the body. One way of telling if your body is saturated with mercury is to have a hair analysis done by a reputable lab such as Doctor's Data in Texas (800-323-2784) or Balco in California (800-777-7122). This test is not fail safe, however. If you are a sensitive person even test results "within normal limits" may mean that there is mercury toxicity in your system.

I recommend three books on the subject of amalgam fillings: *Dental Mercury Detox* and *Dentistry Without Mercury* (Bio-Prove, 1995) by Sam Ziff and Michael F. Ziff, and *It's All in Your Head* (Group West, 1993) by Hal Huggins.

CHAPTER 9: AN HERB AND FIBER CLEANSING PROGRAM

FOS Probiotic Growth Complex

Ultra Flora Plus is available in regular and dairy free forms for the dairy sensitive person. In order to find someone in your area who carries these products, call Metagenics at 800-692-9400 or in Canada at 905-891-1300.

CHAPTER 10: THERAPEUTIC FOOD POWDERS FOR CLEANSING

For information about these products see information in Chapter 9 above.

CHAPTER 11: CLEANSING THE LIVER AND THE LYMPH SYSTEM

Liver Cleansing

Dr. Elson Haas has written about liver-cleansing in his book, *Staying Healthy with the Seasons.* You may utilize his book for further guidance.

The liver cleansing properties of Milk thistle, also called Silymarin, are available in tincture, tablet, and capsule forms in health food stores or by calling 888-85-HEALTH.

Detoxification Factors (Tyler Encapsulations) can be found in doctor's offices or call customer service at 800-869-9705. If they are unable to help, then call 888-85-HEALTH.

Cleansing the Lymph

Adopted by Applied Kinesiology, information on Chapmans' Reflexes can be found in the book *Touch for Health* (DeVorss and Company, 1995) by Dr. John Thie.

For more information, see Charles Owen's compila-
tion "An Endocrine Interpretation of Chapmans' Reflexes"
from the *American Academy of Osteopathy* 1992.

CHAPTER 13: DIET AND RECIPES THAT COMPLEMENT CLEANSING

Nutrition

If you would like to study nutrition in greater depth, Health
Coach offers an excellent video series called *The Diet Health
Connection*. It is a six-part series covering the fundamentals,
important distinctions to consider concerning water, proteins, carbohydrates, lipids, fats, and oils, plus the cholesterol controversy and the role of micronutrients. To enhance
your learning, Dr. Percival and his team created *The Diet
Health Connection Workbook* to accompany the videos. It
increases your ability to remember information up to eighty
percent if you answer questions and write down your
responses. You can order the videos and workbook by calling 800-463-2701.

Cleansing Diet

Dr. Jeffrey Bland has written a book called *The 20 Day Rejuvenation Diet Program* (New Canaan, CT: Keats, 1997) with Sara
Benum, M.A. In this helpful book, Dr. Bland offers an easy-
to-follow holistic prescription for turning around the "walking
wounded" syndrome, wherein you don't feel well but the doctors say nothing is wrong and/or the prescribed medical interventions are not helpful for turning your symptoms around.

Bland outlines a diet program that uses specific foods to counteract metabolic poisons and simultaneously provides the correct balance of nutrients needed by your body. Foods high in beta-carotene and vitamin C are central to the 20 Day Rejuvenation regime. Dr. Bland supplies a shopping list and daily menus (complete with recipes) for readers to follow. He also suggests a regular exercise routine, as physical activity helps eliminate toxics. Packed with personal stories, case studies, and self-evaluation quizzes, *The 20 Day Rejuvenation Diet Program* is for anyone who's trying to recapture physical and psychological zest. Based on clinical experience with thousands of patients who experienced significant health improvement, this consumer-oriented program uses specific rejuvenation foods and phytonutrients in a diet plan carefully designed to prevent problems of accelerated aging and to enhance your energy and vitality. Call them at 800-843-9660.

CHAPTER 14: SUPPLEMENTS TO SUPPORT CLEANSING

Detoxification Tea

You can purchase this delicious combination of gently cleansing and nutritive herbs by calling Mountain Wild Herbals at 800-789-2496.

In Case of Oxidative Stress: Nutrients to Quench Free Radicals

If you have oxidative stress, what are some solutions? In doctors' offices you can purchase Oxygenics, a complete relay team of nutrients to quench free radicals. Many companies have developed antioxidant formulas. The best ones, like Oxygenics, will contain taurine, n-acetyl cysteine, glutathione, and lipoic acid for special support of phase II detoxification in your liver.

Most of the phytonutrients named in Chapter 13 are available in a product called PhytoPro by Metagenics. Although it can't replace whole foods such as fruits, vegetables, nuts, seeds, grains and legumes, PhytoPro can offer a helping hand. If you don't always eat as well as you would like this would be an excellent supplement for your nutritional support program. It comes in powdered or tiny pill form. Find suppliers of Oxygenics, PhytoPro, and Probioplex Intensive Care, by calling Metagenics at 800-692-9400.

CHAPTER 15: PRACTICES THAT COMPLEMENT CLEANSING

Behavioral Change Instruction

If you have a conflict between managing your career and managing your health, Stephen Covey's audio tape or book *Principle Centered Leadership* (New York: Simon and Schuster Trade, 1992) can help you to prioritize what is important to you.

Anthony Robbins is a master at helping people to change limiting behaviors and patterns. Following are descriptions of audiotapes that will help you be the person you want to be. *The Power of Questions* helps you to ask better questions. Mr. Robbins teaches that your questions determine your focus and your focus becomes your reality. *Six Master Steps to Change* teaches you a formula for change that really works. *Creating a Change and Making It Last* guides you through steps to support and reward constructive change. In the final audio, *The Power of Life's Metaphors,* Anthony Robbins teaches you a fascinating and enjoyable way to see how you actually cause yourself problems in all areas of your life by the way you describe your "problems" and how to change your metaphors to support well-being. These tools are available through Health Coach by calling 800-463-2701.

Exercise

Another great resource for health and vitality, including movement, is *The Power of Five: Hundreds of 5-Second to 5-Minute Scientific Shortcuts to Ignite Your Energy, Burn Fat, Stop Aging and Revitalize Your Love Life* (Rodale Press, Emmaus, PA: 1995) by Harold Bloomfield, M.D., and Robert Cooper, Ph.D. Their subtitle best describes what is offered in this useful guide.

Deep Breathing

A recent book, called *The Tao of Natural Breathing* (Associate Publishing, 1996) by Dennis Lewis, emphasizes breathing with the whole body. Here's a quote from an article by Dennis about his new book: "I began to understand that superficial breathing ensures a superficial experience of ourselves, whereas natural breathing opens us to our own inner spaces and to the energies of the universe."

Rest and Relaxation

Journey to Health, by Larry Herdener, N.D., guides you through the process of progressive relaxation as well as special meditations to assist your cleansing program. This tape may be purchased by calling 888-85-HEALTH.

If you would like to contact The Healing Tao Center for information, a catalog of books, or a referral to an instructor in your area, please write: The Healing Tao Center, P.O. Box 1194, Huntington, N.Y. 11743.

The Inner Smile

"The Inner Smile" is available on a two-sided audiocassette by calling 888-85-HEALTH (888-854-3258). Side one guides you through a process of bringing healing energy into your organs, digestive system, and spine, then into every system and cell in your body. Side two has two shorter healing exercises. "Smile into Your Distress" assists you in dissolving the hold that stressful situations have on you. The second one, "Smile into Ecstasy," increases the joy in your mind, body, and heart.

APPENDIX 2: INFANT CARE

Infant Nutrition

If you would like to read more about feeding your infant nourishing foods that will keep, you can purchase the book *Infant Nutrition* by Mark Percival, D.C., N.D., from Health Coach Systems International by calling 800-463-2701.

Metagenics has an excellent, well tolerated (even in the first trimester of pregnancy when some women are experiencing nausea) prenatal supplement available through doctors' offices.

APPENDIX 2: INFANT CARE

Even commercial baby's milk is "rich" in toxic materials. If you choose not to breast-feed your infant or need to supplement with formula, please heed the following recommendations.

Stay away from premixed formula in cans. There is a high likelihood that the cans are coated inside with a plastic resin. You don't want to expose your little one to that hormone-altering material.

Read the ingredients. When I was doing some research in my local drug store, I was surprised to find that sugar was included in some of the formulas. Corn syrup was the first ingredient in one of the nondairy formulas. All of them contained vegetable oil (see Essential Fatty Acids in Appendix 3). What I have said in this book about commercial vegetable oils—the way they have been produced and the damaging effects they can have on a body—should raise a red flag of warning. There are no "good" substitutes for a mother's milk.

Carnation Good Start may be your baby's best option if you cannot breast-feed. The sweetener is lactose, instead of sugar or corn syrup, which is healthier unless the infant has a lactose intolerance. The protein comes from *lactalbumin* (a milk protein) which has been partially digested, making it less allergenic.

To compensate for nutrition lacking in a formula, you can supplement feedings with some of the products mentioned in this book, especially flaxseed oil and/or DHA and bifidobacteria. With respect to the flaxseed oil, for the first ten pounds of body weight ¼ teaspoon per day will do; you can feed your baby the fresh oil on a spoon or rub twice as much directly onto its skin. For ten to eighteen pounds of body weight use ½ teaspoon; at twenty-six to thirty-five pounds use ¾ teaspoon; and above thirty-five pounds use 1 teaspoon for each thirty-five pounds of body weight.

It may be safer and more effective to use the DHA product "Neuramins" produced by Martek in this situation (see Appendix 1). Neuramins is an omega-3 EFA concentrate made from an ocean algae source. The best way for baby to get this important nutrient is from the mother. Unfortunately, because of changes in our diet, mothers now have only half the level of DHA they had fifty years ago. EFAs from flaxseed oil and/or DHA are needed for the optimal development of your baby's brain and eyes. Other body tissues that have a high concentration of DHA are the heart, liver, and semen. DHA also supports immune system function and the health of baby's skin. The World Health Organization recommends approximately ten milligrams of DHA for every pound of body weight. So a ten-pound baby would need a minimum of approximately eighty milligrams of this EFA.

There is scientific evidence that the DHA the mother takes crosses the placenta to nourish her baby's brain. Martek recommends that pregnant and lactating moms take 200 mg of Neuramins each day since they are feeding half their supply to the fetus or newborn. Neuramins will be available soon in large retail stores such as Wal-Mart at a very reasonable price, according to one of the company founders. You may also be able to purchase it through a doctor's office that is on the cutting edge of nutritional science. If you are unable to find DHA, you may order it by calling 888-85-HEALTH.

In Europe and Asia, all infant formulas are supplemented with DHA. Why don't American babies get the same consideration? International studies going back twenty to thirty years show a dose-dependent response with respect to the DHA content in baby's pre- and post-natal diets. That means that the greater the dose of DHA, the greater the response in terms of visual acuity and mental development as measured by the Mental Development Index. Infants who were breast-fed for up to eight months showed linear improvement in long-term development up to nine years of age.

Mother's milk is high in bifidobacteria, which demonstrates immune-supportive effects. You can read more about this and about nourishing probiotic formulas in Chapter 14. I would recommend using probiotics only from Metagenics because of the care they take to ensure the purity and efficacy of their products. In doctor's offices, you can find bifidobacteria in a product called Ultra Bifidus. If your baby is dairy-sensitive you can purchase this product in a dairy-free version. Use ¼ teaspoon three times per day. If you are breast-feeding but your newborn still needs an extra immune-system boost, you can make the powder into a paste with a little water and rub it onto your nipple for your baby to eat while he or she nurses. If you are using formula, mix it right in the bottle. The bifidobacteria must be refrigerated.

If your infant is not dairy-sensitive you can also add Probioplex Intensive Care (Metagenics). This product is especially good for normalizing diarrhea. Give your child half the adult dose: ½ tablespoon one to two times per day.

These products are not harmful in any way as long as you follow the mentioned precaution with a dairy-sensitive infant. They will only add to your baby's health and well-being. Probioplex Intensive Care has the advantage of not needing refrigeration.

Don't worry about mixing up these recommendations. It tells you what to do right on the label, except that the dose for your infant is half of the adult dose. Remember: although your baby does not weigh half of what an adult weighs, if you were breast-feeding, your baby would be getting these nutrients in large quantities from breast milk. Proportionately, babies need a larger amount than adults because of their developing digestive and immune systems. Acidophilus supplements will be of no use to your baby until the baby is two-and-one-half to three years old. (To purchase Metagenics products, call 800-692-9400 to find a health care practitioner who carries them in your area.)

Appendix 3: Essential Fatty Acids and Omega-3 Supplements

I have taken flaxseed oil for a long time, but until reading *The Omega 3 Phenomenon* and speaking to Fred Rohe and reading his book *Eat Fat: Your Life Depends on It,* I was taking too little for my weight. For the past three weeks, I have increased my dosage and have been amazed by the changes I have so far enjoyed. The dry skin on the back of my arms, which manifested as little rough spots by the hair follicles, has become softer, smoother, and more silky to the touch. I notice that I remember phone numbers better when I am calling someone; I don't have to look at the number twice to complete dialing. My muscles feel stronger, and I am more stable on my feet; I haven't been leaning against the chiropractic table so much when working on patients. And I am waking up earlier with a clear head, feeling rested. The proper dose of flaxseed oil has already added considerable value and zest to my life.

Health Benefits of EFAs

In their book, *The Omega-3 Phenomenon,* Dr. Donald Rudin and Clara Felix outline the benefits of omega-3 fatty acid supplements:

1. Skin improvements such as softer, smoother, firmer, flawless skin with improved tone and color, reduced sun sensitivity, and some fading of age spots on the hands.
2. Shinier, thicker, fuller hair.
3. Vitality, a zest for life, and increased stamina that lasts for long periods of time.
4. Smoother muscle action leading to greater agility.
5. Elimination of bingeing and the addictive need for food.
6. Reduction or elimination of food allergies.
7. Improved resistance to some diseases.
8. Improved functioning of the digestive tract, avoiding gas, constipation, and other disorders.
9. Stronger cardiovascular system.
10. Increased fat metabolism.
11. Clearer thinking.
12. Increased resistance to cold weather.
13. Increased physical comfort.
14. Improved quality of life.

Felix and Rudin say that if you include omega-3 fatty acid supplements in your daily diet, you can expect benefits in as little as two hours; in some cases, improvement may continue for one or two years before leveling off.

Felix and Rudin did not include information in their list about the anti-carcinogenic effects of taking a flaxseed oil supplement. More recent research shows that omega-3 fatty acids kill human cancer cells in tissue cultures without destroying the normal cells in the same cultures. Breast, lung, and prostate cancer cells were studied. Omega-3 fatty acids lower high blood pressure and triglyceride levels. They decrease the probability of a blood clot blocking an artery in the brain (causing a stroke), in the heart (causing a heart attack), in the lungs (causing a pulmonary embolism), or in other organs (causing peripheral vascular disease such as gangrene).

The study by J.J.F. Belch titled "Effects of Altering Dietary Essential Fatty Acids on Requirements for Non-Steroidal Anti-Inflammatory Drugs in Patients with Rheumatoid Arthritis" (*Annals of Rheumatic Diseases*, 1988) showed that by using a combination of the omega-3 and omega-6 fatty acids, rheumatoid arthritics were able to completely discontinue or decrease their *nonsteroidal anti-inflammatory drugs* (NSAIDs), such as aspirin, Tylenol, ibuprofen, and Motrin. This is a very good thing, because NSAIDs inhibit your liver's ability to process poisons from food, water, air, perfumes, colognes, body lotions, potions, and creams that you come into contact with or that you put on your skin on a regular basis. According to a November 1, 1995, article in *Family Practice News*, "One-fifth of all drug reactions reported to the Food and Drug Administration involved NSAIDs."

THE IMPORTANCE OF BALANCED EFAs

Much of the information about fatty acids shared here comes from discussions with Fred Rohe and from reading his book, *Eat Fat: Your Life Depends on It*. Rohe discusses the optimal balance between omega-6 and omega-3 EFAs. Experts vary in their opinion of what is the best ratio. The ratio in your body tissue is 4:1, except in the brain and sex glands, where it is 1:1. The Standard American Diet (SAD) is grossly imbalanced, with a ratio of between 10:1 and 20:1.

Your body has different needs at different times, so it is impossible to always be perfect about the ratio of EFAs that you consume. Rohe recommends eating a variety of oils and taking an EFA supplement with a good average ratio of omega-6: omega-3 EFAs to insure an adequate supply of EFAs for most people most of the time. Children need EFAs, too. To encourage brain development, use a 1:1 ratio until puberty.

- For a 1:1 ratio, mix 3 parts fresh flaxseed oil with 2 parts fresh sunflower oil.
- For a 2:1 ratio, mix 1 part fresh flaxseed oil with 2 parts fresh sunflower oil.
- For a 3:1 ratio, mix 1 part fresh flaxseed oil with 3 parts fresh sunflower oil.

Remember, though, that you are probably starting with an imbalanced fatty acid status. If a core sample of your fat could be taken, it would tell you just what type of fats you have been eating. Since most fats and oils in the marketplace are trans fats, which are destroyed by processing or hydrogenation, you are probably severely deficient in EFAs—especially omega-3. A period of supplementation with fresh flaxseed oil exclusively, which is in a 1:3 omega-6 to omega-3 ratio, while eliminating *trans* fats from your diet, will help to improve your body fat constitution and your health. Continue with the flaxseed oil alone for three to six months. If you continue to eat a significant amount of omega-6 oils by eating out a lot or consuming quantities of sunflower or sesame seeds or any other oil than flaxseed oil, you may need to continue with fresh flaxseed oil with its 1:3 ratio over the long term.

BUY HIGH-QUALITY OILS

In order to ensure that you are eating only high-quality oils, look for oils that:

- are processed below 118°F
- are processed excluding light and air
- are processed without toxic solvents
- are bottled in opaque containers
- have air displaced by inert gas

Fats are altered not only by the processes mentioned above, but also by the normal processing that all but a few brands undergo. Oils, even those sold in health food stores, are expeller-pressed, with presses the size of railroad cars subjecting them to temperatures of up to 180°F, and filtration through phosphates and caustic sodas. Bleach deodorizing further raises the temperature to 520°F. If the oil is produced by a large commercial company, it will also be run through a solvent extraction using hexane—a volatile liquid paraffin hydrocarbon found in petroleum—to increase the oil yield and their profits. Expeller-pressed "natural brands" undergo the same process, minus the hexane treatment. They may even call this oil "cold-pressed" because there are no regulations about what "cold-pressed" means. The end product—the oil you buy at the market—has minimal nutritional value and little similarity to real food. Nutrients are either altered or removed and, to amplify this transgression against human health and well-being, it contains poisonous *trans* fatty acids, free radicals, and other toxic substances. Periodic cleansing, supplemental nutrients, and high-quality oils help to prevent the damage of this now-unavoidable material, commercially processed vegetable oils.

EFAs are sensitive to damage from heat and light, which is why it is important to process them below 118°F and to store them in opaque containers. Opaque plastic is the material of choice for those companies that produce fresh oils. Most oil is sold in clear or tinted glass bottles, which exposes them to enough light to change their chemical composition, producing toxic, cancer-causing substances. The metal tins in which much olive oil is stored also damage the oil. The solder that holds their seams together is probably made from tin and lead—not optimal for contact with your food.

APPENDIX 4:
TESTS AND SELF EXAMS

TEST YOUR pH LEVEL

The pH of each portion of the GI tract is critical for the activation of the various digestive juices. The mouth and *esophagus* — the tube running between your mouth and stomach — optimally maintain a neutral pH of 7.0 to 7.2. You can check the pH of your own mouth with litmus paper. You can also use litmus paper to perform the following simple experiment, which will indicate whether you have a "health reserve."

1. Put a small piece of litmus paper (ordering instructions follow) in your mouth and determine the pH by comparing the color against the color chart on the litmus paper container.
2. Cut off a slice of fresh lemon and suck out all of the juice.
3. Swish the juice around in your mouth, then swallow it.
4. Wait one minute (sixty seconds).
5. Retest your pH by placing another piece of litmus paper in your mouth.
6. Compare your pH to the pH you noted before sucking the lemon.

Has your pH increased, stayed the same, or dropped relative to your original reading? Your findings can be likened to a financial portfolio. If your pH stayed the same, it's like living from day to day and having only enough money to cover your expenses. If your pH increases above the optimal range, you have "savings" to increase your current well-being and security in times of stress. On the other hand, if your pH dropped below optimal, you are running up your "debts" and moving toward "bankruptcy" unless you begin to make some significant changes.

You can get litmus paper from your local pharmacy or order it direct from:

Micro Essential Nutrients
4224 Avenue H
Brooklyn, NY 11210
Phone: 718-388-3618
Fax: 718-692-4491

TEST YOUR LEVEL OF STOMACH AND OTHER DIGESTIVE ACIDS

The next portion of your GI tract, your stomach, must be acidic or have a very low pH to stimulate the more alkaline secretions of your small intestine. If your stomach acids are weak there is no impetus for your body to produce strong alkaline or basic enzymes.

To determine if your digestive secretions are low, observe whether and when you get gas following a meal. Gas soon after eating is a sign that your stomach secretions are low. If you get gas within an hour or two after eating, your small intestine's digestion is probably deficient. A Health Coach can help you assess the state of your digestion by taking a history, completing a thorough physical examination, and reviewing questionnaires that you have filled out prior to your visit. Or else try the service of a gastroenterologist.

Laboratory tests are also available but are more invasive and costly. The Heidelberg test for adequate stomach secretions is performed by placing a capsule down your throat and esophagus into your stomach. The capsule acts as a battery, and a receiver in the room where the test is conducted picks up information from the capsule and measures your stomach acidity or lack thereof. An osteopath friend who conducts the test says that the procedure can sometimes take two hours. At least one of my colleagues believes that this test is inaccurate because having an object stuck down your throat and into your stomach puts you into an alarm state that shuts down your digestive juices.

The final portion of your intestines, the colon, may also be evaluated for a variety of markers such as pH which are indicative of health or disease through stool analysis. This is a valuable test done by many progressive doctors, and you do have to go through the process of collecting the stool sample and sending it off to the lab in a timely manner so that the results will be accurate. I recommend Great Smokies Diagnostic Laboratory (GSDL) in Asheville, North Carolina. After carefully analyzing six tons of samples last year, they have established themselves as the leaders in the field of stool analysis and functional body assessment tests. You may reach them by calling 800-522-4762 and asking for customer service. They will be happy to put you in touch with a licensed health care professional in your area who uses this technology.

TEST YOUR LIVER FUNCTION

If you would like to find out how your liver is functioning, contact GSDL. One of the nice things about GSDL's stool test is that they check to see which pharmaceutical drugs and natural herbal substances destroy the harmful microorganisms found in your stool sample. Many of the findings in their Complete Digestive Stool Analysis measure your level of protective substances against cancer of the breast, prostate, and colon compared to what would be found in a healthy person. Since these cancers are great killers in our population, it makes sense to find out where you stand if you want to live a healthy, vibrant life. If the profile doesn't look good, you can then get some good advice from a natural health care professional or make necessary changes on your own, such as the ones recommended in *Internal Cleansing,* to restore your vibrant health.

TEST YOUR LEVEL OF OXIDATIVE STRESS

Oxidative Stress Questionnaire

Point Scale

> 0 = None or Never
> 1 = Slight or Rarely
> 2 = Mild or Occasionally
> 3 = Moderate or Frequently
> 4 = Severe or Almost Always

Answer each of the following questions relative to your symptoms or history over the past month. Once you've completed the questionnaire, ask a Health Coach or seek a health care practitioner who can help you interpret the results.

1. ___ Do you have symptoms that are aggravated by air pollution?
2. ___ Are you sensitive to smoke, perfume, or other chemical odors?
3. ___ Do you have ongoing problems with fatigue?

4. ___ Do suffer from joint pain or deep muscle pain?
5. ___ Do you have a significant environmental exposure to pollutants (at work or at home)?
6. ___ Rate your use of tobacco products.
7. ___ Rate your exposure to second-hand smoke.
8. ___ Rate your consumption of alcoholic beverages.
9. ___ Rate your unprotected exposure to sunlight or ultraviolet light.
10. ___ Rate your level of exercise.
11. ___ What is your exposure to prescription drugs, over-the-counter medications, and/or recreational drugs?
12. ___ Rate your daily stress level.
13. ___ Rate your intake of fried foods, margarine, or high-fat foods.
14. ___ How often do you seek medical care or advice for your health concerns?

Add up the numbers to arrive at a total.
   ___ Total
   ___ Are you currently taking antioxidant supplements?
   ___ Yes   ___ No

Reprinted by permission of HealthComm International, Inc.

In addition to the Oxidative Stress Questionnaire, objective laboratory tests can be performed to evaluate whether you are at risk for damage to your heart, lungs, gastrointestinal tract, or nervous system from free radicals. You can also call GSDL, which can measure the amount of oxidative stress in your body using blood and urine tests.

BIBLIOGRAPHY

Ashley, Cynthia, and Sylvia Valazques. *Creative Reuse Extravaganza.* Oakland, CA: East Bay Depot for Creative Reuse, Inc., 1996.

Blair, Steven. *Living with Exercise.* Dallas, TX: American Health Publishing Company, 1991.

Bland, Ph.D., Jeffrey. *The 20-Day Rejuvenation Diet Program.* New Canaan, CT: Keats Publishing, 1997.

Borman, Herbert. F., Diana Balmori, and Gordon T. Geballe. *Redesigning the American Lawn.* New Haven and London: Yale University Press, 1993.

Colborn, Theo, Dianne Dumanoski, and John Peterson Myers. *Our Stolen Future.* New York: Dutton, 1997.

Covey, Steven. *First Things First.* New York: Simon and Schuster, 1994.

Erasmus, Udo. *Fats That Heal, Fats That Kill.* Blaine, WA: Alive Books, 1993.

Finnegan, John. *The Facts About Fats.* Berkeley, CA: Celestial Arts, 1993.

Jensen, Bernard. *Tissue Cleansing Through Bowel Management.* Escondido, CA: Bernard Jensen Enterprises, 1981.

Kapit, Wynn, and Lawrence M. Elson. *The Anatomy Coloring Book.* New York: Harper College Publishers, 1993.

O'Regan, Brendan, and Caryle Hirshberg. *Spontaneous Remission: An Annotated Bibliography.* Sausalito, CA: Institute of Noetic Sciences, 1995.

Owen, Charles. *An Endocrine Interpretation of Chapman's Reflexes.* Newark, Ohio: American Academy of Osteopathy, 1992.

Percival, D.C., N.D., Mark. *Infant Nutrition.* New Hamburg, Ontario: Health Coach Systems International, 1994.

Percival, D.C., N.D., Mark. *Functional Dietetics: The Core of Health Integration.* New Hamburg, Ontario: Health Coach Systems International, 1995.

Percival, D.C., N.D., Mark, and Cheri Percival. *Guilt Free Indulgence: A Cookbook with Conscience.* New Hamburg, Ontario: Health Coach Systems International, 1995.

Rudin, M.D., Donald O., and Clara Felix. *The Omega 3 Phenomenon.* New York: Rawson Associates, 1987.

Rudin M.D., Donald O., and Clara Felix. *Omega 3 Oils to Improve Mental Health, Fight Degenerative Diseases, and Extend Your Life.* Garden City Park, NY: Avery Publishing, 1996.

Samuels, M.D., Mike, and Hal Zina Bennett. *Well Body, Well Earth.* San Francisco: Sierra Club Books, 1985.

Siguel, M.D., Edward. *Essential Fatty Acids in Health and Disease.* Boston, MA: Boston University Medical Center. 1994.

Thie, John. *Touch for Health.* Marina del Ray, CA: DeVorss and Company. 1995.

INDEX

GETTING WELL NATURALLY SERIES

Michael T. Murray, N.D.

In the highly successful GETTING WELL NATURALLY series, natural medicine researcher Dr. Michael T. Murray shares his extensive knowledge of herbs, exercise, and other natural healing methods with health conscious readers. Dr. Murray's popular books help you understand and control chronic health problems and promote whole-body physical and emotional wellness. Each volume in the series provides natural programs, specific courses of treatment, dietary guidelines, and the latest information on a wide range of conditions.

Arthritis
ISBN 1-55958-491-2 / paperback
176 pages
U.S. $9.95 / Can. $13.95

Male Sexual Vitality
ISBN 1-55958-428-9 / paperback
160 pages
U.S. $10.95 / Can. $14.95

Chronic Candidiasis
ISBN 0-7615-0821-X / paperback
192 pages
U.S. $11.00 / Can. $14.95

Menopause
ISBN 1-55958-427-0 / paperback
192 pages
U.S. $12.95 / Can. $17.95

Chronic Fatigue Syndrome
ISBN 1-55958-490-4 / paperback
208 pages
U.S. $11.00 / Can. $14.95

Premenstrual Syndrome
ISBN 0-7615-0820-1 / paperback
176 pages
U.S. $11.00 / Can. $14.95

Diabetes & Hypoglycemia
ISBN 1-55958-426-2 / paperback
176 pages
U.S. $9.95 / Can. $14.95

Stomach Ailments and Digestive Disturbances
ISBN 0-7615-0657-8 / paperback
208 pages
U.S. $11.00 / Can. $14.95

Heart Disease and High Blood Pressure
ISBN 0-7615-0658-6 / paperback
192 pages
U.S. $11.00 / Can. $14.95

Stress, Anxiety & Insomnia
ISBN 1-55958-489-0 / paperback
192 pages
U.S. $11.00 / Can. $14.95

Herbal Prescriptions for Better Health

Your Up-to-Date Guide to the Most Effective
Herbal Treatments

Donald J. Brown, N.D.

U.S. $16.00
Can. $21.95
ISBN: 0-7615-1001-X
paperback / 368 pages

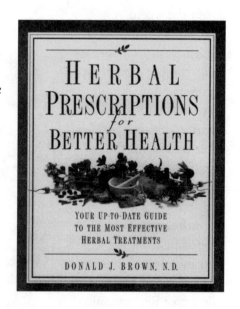

Let nature's own remedies work for you! Here's an indispensable guide that introduces you to effective and safe ways to improve your health through the power of herbal medicines. In this insightful book, Dr. Donald Brown recommends specific herbal treatments for dozens of common ailments and provides answers to frequently asked questions. From herbs such as aloe vera, feverfew, ginseng, and goldenseal, you'll find solutions for numerous health conditions, including those related to the heart, digestive system, skin, urinary tract, and more!

Living Foods for Optimum Health

A Highly Effective Program to Remove Toxins and Restore Your Body to Vibrant Health

Brian R. Clement
with Theresa Foy DiGeronimo

U.S. $22.95
Can. $29.95
ISBN 0-7615-0258-0
hardcover / 288 pages

From the world-renowned Hippocrates Health Institute, here is your complete guide to the miraculous healing potential of raw foods. Learn to cleanse and heal your body with the naturally potent, fresh, organic, unrefined foods that have enabled countless people to overcome life-threatening illnesses such as cancer and heart disease or heal chronic ailments such as asthma and arthritis. Including the why and how of a living-foods lifestyle and more than 100 healthful, delicious recipes, this book lets you take personal control of your health and well-being.

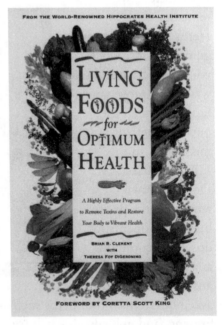

Eat Your Way to Better Health

*Good Health and Great Recipes with the
Superpyramid Eating Program*

Dr. Gene Spiller

U.S. $16.00
Can. $21.95
ISBN 0-7615-0617-9
paperback / 528 pages

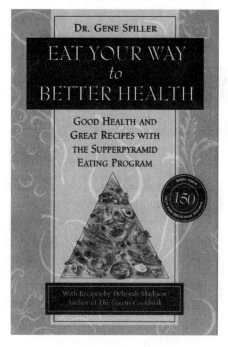

You don't have to confine yourself to a merciless dietary regime, you don't have to count calories, and you don't have to give up good food. Founded on the enjoyment and celebration of food, this book combines the knowledge of a leading nutritionist with more than 150 great recipes from master chef Deborah Madison to bring you a practical, reasonable, easy program for total fitness and overall well-being. Here is a pyramid path to better health that invites you to revel in the natural bounty of wholesome real foods without the number crunching of servings, serving sizes, calorie counts, or grams of fat. Enjoy the best the Earth has to offer!

To Order Books

Please send me the following items:

Quantity	Title	Unit Price	Total
_____	_____	$ _____	$ _____
_____	_____	$ _____	$ _____
_____	_____	$ _____	$ _____
_____	_____	$ _____	$ _____
_____	_____	$ _____	$ _____

Shipping and Handling depend on Subtotal.

Subtotal	Shipping/Handling
$0.00–$14.99	$3.00
$15.00–$29.99	$4.00
$30.00–$49.99	$6.00
$50.00–$99.99	$10.00
$100.00–$199.99	$13.50
$200.00+	Call for Quote

Foreign and all Priority Request orders:
Call Order Entry department
for price quote at 916/632-4400

This chart represents the total retail price of books only (before applicable discounts are taken).

Subtotal $ _____

Deduct 10% when ordering 3-5 books $ _____

7.25% Sales Tax (CA only) $ _____

8.25% Sales Tax (TN only) $ _____

5.0% Sales Tax (MD and IN only) $ _____

Shipping and Handling* $ _____

Total Order $ _____

By Telephone: With MC or Visa, call 800-632-8676 or 916-632-4400.
Mon–Fri, 8:30-4:30.

WWW: http://www.primapublishing.com

By Internet E-mail: sales@primapub.com

By Mail: Just fill out the information below and send with your remittance to:

**Prima Publishing
P.O. Box 1260BK
Rocklin, CA 95677**

My name is _____

I live at _____

City _____ State _____ ZIP_____

MC/Visa#_____ Exp. _____

Check/money order enclosed for $_____ Payable to Prima Publishing

Daytime telephone _____

Signature _____